T0129363

The Reiki Magic Guide
to Self-Attunement

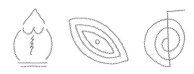

The Reiki Magic Guide
to Self-Attunement

Brett Bevell

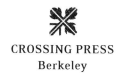

CROSSING PRESS
Berkeley

Healing and medicine are two very different disciplines and the law
requires the following disclaimer: The information in this book is not medicine but healing, and does not constitute medical advice. In case of serious
illness consult your practitioner of choice.

Published in the United States by Crossing Press, an imprint of the Crown
Publishing Group, a division of Random House, Inc., New York.
www.crownpublishing.com
www.tenspeed.com

Crossing Press and the Crossing Press colophon are registered trademarks of
Random House, Inc.

Library of Congress Cataloging-in-Publication Data
Bevell, Brett.
The Reiki magic guide to self-attunement / Brett Bevell.
        p. cm.
Includes index.
1. Reiki (Healing system) I. Title.

RZ403.R45B48 2007
615.8'52—dc22

                    2007008250

ISBN 978-1-58091-184-9

Cover design by Alan Hebel
Text design by Michael Cutter
Reiki self-treatment illustrations by Ann Miya
Back cover author photo by Jan Campbell

First Edition

146086900

For Helema Kadir, and all who are working for world peace.

Contents

Acknowledgments

I OWE GRATITUDE TO Pan, Jesus, the Goddess Sekhmet, Ra Ta (Edgar Cayce), and the Deva of Reiki for inspiring and guiding me through this process. I owe gratitude as well to Ric Weinman, founder of VortexHealing® Divine Energy Healing, and Merlin (the Avatar), the source of the VortexHealing lineage, for adding a VortexHealing energetic upgrade to what was already an effective process of Reiki attunement made available to all who read this book. And I deeply wish to thank my shaman friend Carolion, and fellow Reiki Masters Hethyrre, Michele Denis, and Noelle Adamo for all their support, advice, and encouragement, as well as for allowing me to experiment on them and with them over the past decade.

Introduction

THE BOOK YOU HOLD in your hands is magical. Magic in esoteric terms is the focusing of mental, psychic, or spiritual energy through ritual, prayer, or other means to effect outcomes in our lives that are in accordance with our personal will or Divine will. The word *magic* also connotes a sense of wonder, as in *having a magical childhood.* This book is magical because if used properly it will enhance that sense of wonder in your life, and take your consciousness to the furthest reaches imaginable. Most importantly, however, this book is magical because it has a unique power, the power to connect you to Reiki attunements that have been sent through the time/space matrix. These attunements are as eternal lines of light, existing through time, and can be intersected and invoked by repeated sacred words offered in this text. The attunement process offered through this book has been refined and researched since 1995, and has proven to be as effective as an in-person Reiki attunement. Many will question both the technique and ethics of this book. It is revolutionary, and thus breaks down barriers that presently are comfortable for some, barriers that also prevent the mass awakening of humanity to this wonderful and easily accessible gift called Reiki. The potential exists to make Reiki a part of our daily lives and a common aspect of human living, to bring Reiki into our homes, into our food and water, into almost every aspect of our being. I have written *The Reiki Magic Guide to Self-Attunement* to see Reiki evolve beyond simply being a healing tool offered in privately paid for sessions, and become instead a commonly understood aspect of our existence, which unfolds toward an even greater awakening of our potential as peaceful spiritual beings taking ownership of our spiritual inheritance. This book presents one possible pathway toward this goal.

1

Reiki Lineage and Evolution

Reiki is a form of hands-on energy healing that comes from the Divine. It is an intelligent healing energy that flows through anyone who has received a Reiki initiation, which is called an attunement. Once a person is attuned to Reiki, he or she has the ability to use this energy for healing themselves or others, an ability that remains for an entire lifetime. Some often confuse Reiki with psychic energy, which it is not. If you were to think of it in terms of a form of radiation, psychic energy radiates from each of us individually, whereas Reiki radiates from the Divine, but is allowed to flow through people who are initiated into the Reiki lineage. Thus, Reiki has an intelligence as well as compassion and a healing quality much greater than that of any individual human being. It is as limitless as the Divine source from which it comes. During Reiki sessions, the energy always seems to know where to go and what to do, unlike psychic energy, which needs to be consciously directed. The beautiful thing about the Reiki lineage of healing is that it does not require you to be psychic or intuitive or have any special abilities. Once you are attuned to this sacred energy, all you have to do is desire it to run through your own hands into whomever or whatever you intend to heal.

The First Reiki Master: Dr. Mikao Usui

The present Reiki lineage on this planet began through the efforts of Dr. Mikao Usui, a Japanese healer and the world's first Reiki Master, who lived from 1865 to 1926. Dr. Usui believed that humanity had once had a vast spiritual ability to heal, like the healing performed by Jesus and Buddha that is mentioned in sacred religious texts. His search to rediscover the source of this healing—a search that lasted for approximately seven years—included researching sacred texts, meditating, and eventually praying and fasting on a sacred mountaintop for twenty-one days. At the end of this twenty-one-day period, Dr. Usui had a mystical experience in which he was Divinely blessed with a wonderful healing gift, a gift that Dr. Usui called Reiki, a Japanese word that literally translates as "Universal Life Force." When Dr. Usui received this initiation from the Divine, he saw "bubbles of light" coming down from the heavens, and these "bubbles of light" opened him to be able to flow what he called Reiki out of his hands. Shortly after his mystical experience, Dr. Usui injured his foot while coming down from the mountain where he had been fasting. He placed his hands on his foot and through Reiki healed his injury. From that day forward for the remainder of his life, Dr. Usui pursued a life path of healing in which he used Reiki to heal others, taught Reiki to those interested in learning it, and opened a Reiki clinic where other Reiki Masters were trained so that the lineage could live on after his death.

There is much speculation about the exact history surrounding this mysterious man. Some of what is written about him perhaps is legend, while other elements are truthful. Whether he was a Christian minister (as some books say) or a Buddhist monk (as other sources say) is speculation. What all written sources about Dr. Mikao Usui do confirm is that he was a man engaged on a mystical path who discovered a spiritual source of healing that he called Reiki.

In my own personal experience as a healer and teacher of Reiki, and as one who respects all spiritual traditions, I honor Dr. Mikao Usui for bringing Reiki to this planet, for offering it as a simple yet powerful healing tool that all are capable of learning. What is important is not so much what his own spiritual practices were, but that he went deep enough into them to get close enough to the Source of all things so that he could then bring forward this wonderful healing energy we call Reiki.

There is also speculation about how Dr. Usui taught Reiki during his lifetime. Some say he used the degree system and symbols commonly known in the Reiki system as they are taught today. Others say that he used no symbols, that he had no system of degrees, and that the attunement process was a repeated energy transference that happened over a prolonged period of time via a method referred to as Rei-ju. Again, the real truth seems somewhat shrouded in mystery.

Reiki Spreads Throughout the World

The history of Reiki after Dr. Usui died also has elements of speculation, but what is evident from all sources is that prior to World War II Reiki was brought to America by a Japanese-American woman named Hawayo Takata. She received her training as a Reiki Master in Tokyo in 1938 by Chujiro Hayashi, one of the Reiki Masters initiated by Dr. Usui. Upon leaving Japan, Hawayo Takata began offering Reiki training and healing in the United States, first in Hawaii and eventually in San Francisco. Though Hawayo Takata died in December of 1980, she attuned twenty-two Reiki Masters during her lifetime. These twenty-two Reiki Masters trained and attuned numerous other Reiki students, and the number of Reiki Masters and practitioners has been growing exponentially ever since.

Today Reiki can found in every state of the United States and in most countries around the world. Reiki can now even be found in some progressive hospitals. And in many states, nurses and massage therapists can receive continuing education units for learning this wonderful healing art. The purpose of this book is to expand the role of Reiki even more, so that Reiki becomes a common aspect of the human experience and available to all people who wish for it.

My Experience with Reiki

My own experience with Reiki began back in 1992 after getting my tooth pulled at NYU Dental School. My gums were killing me, and my roommate, Eben, told me he thought he could help me by placing his hands on my cheek and doing an energy healing I had not yet heard of, called Reiki. My mouth was swollen, as the dental student who had pulled my wisdom tooth had been very rough. I was in pain, and nothing seemed to help the swelling go down. But when Eben placed his hands on my cheek I felt a sense of relief. It was not that all the pain went away. It didn't go away entirely. But I did have a sense of relief, a sense that I was loved by some power much greater than myself. And this sensation of love was coming through Eben's hands as he performed the Reiki treatment on me. I was soothed, and felt like suddenly

I was bigger than the pain, that I would outlast the pain. And I felt that eventually I would heal. Further into the session, I began to feel sleepy. And when the treatment ended thirty minutes later I had a deep sense of calm that filled my entire being.

That was my introduction to Reiki. No words could have explained to me what this fabulous energy was, or what it could do for me. I had to experience it directly. I did not know then that one day I would become a Reiki practitioner, or that I would go on to become a Reiki Master. But I had been touched by a gentle loving energy, an energy that would change my life. What I did not realize was that this energy had the power to change all of humanity, but that humanity had to experience it directly to really understand it.

My own Reiki training has involved three different Reiki Masters. I received First Degree by Reiki Master Elka Petra Palm, a teacher from the Reiki Alliance, who gave me a solid foundation in the traditional understanding of Reiki; Second Degree by Mary Roberson, a Reiki Master who encouraged me to playfully explore with Reiki as a form of expanding my consciousness; and Master Level Reiki from Reiki Master Mary Dudek, who trained me how to share this gift from a place of simplicity.

The Evolution of Reiki and Human Consciousness

My evolution with Reiki has taught me that the system of Reiki itself is evolving as human consciousness evolves. Where once it may have been extremely important to speak of lineage, to remain tied to how Reiki has been explained to us by others, over the years I have found that the greatest discovery in Reiki comes from listening to the energy itself, taking it out of the realm of personality or dogma. Thus, for many years I simply experimented with how the energy of Reiki could be adapted and used in creative ways. I did not disregard the teachings of my Reiki Masters, but simply saw that there was more to Reiki than anyone had ever explained to me. I also incorporated my knowledge of Machaelle Small Wright's groundbreaking work through her book *MAP: The Co-Creative White Brotherhood Medical Assistance Program*, using her techniques to connect with the Devic realm and receive guidance from the spirit world in how to expand Reiki as a system.

My primary assumption in all my Reiki experiments was that as long as I was not harming anyone or invading anyone's free will, I was free to expand how I used Reiki as guided by my spirit teachers. Over the years, I was shown innovative ways to adapt the Reiki attunement process for absentee attunements, first by sending Reiki attunements into a labyrinth so that anyone who walked that specific labyrinth and asked for an attunement while in the center would be attuned to First Degree Reiki. I asked several friends who were not attuned to Reiki but had an interest to learn Reiki to walk the labyrinth and make the request for an attunement to First Degree Reiki. In each case (which happened over a period of months), when I felt their hands after they had walked the labyrinth and requested the attunement, their hands were flowing Reiki. Later, my spirit teachers showed me that walking the labyrinth was not actually necessary, that the attunement could be sent linked just to a specific phrase, an empowered series of words, and that by simply stating the phrase with right intention one would be attuned to Reiki.

In the summer of 2000, I began teaching Reiki to staff at the world's largest holistic learning center, Omega Institute for Holistic Studies in Rhinebeck, New York. Since 2002, I have been teaching Reiki Master classes to Omega staff as well, and have had many instances where the teachings from this book have been confirmed in classes with my students.

As Shakespeare wrote in his wonderful play *Hamlet*: "There are more things in heaven and earth, Horatio, than are dreamt of in your philosophy." This is true of Reiki as well. Reiki historically has always been shrouded in mystery, and where mystery exists, there is always room to explore the unknown. Let us respect Reiki lineage, but not let it bind us to the ignorance of pretending we know all that is potentially true about this wonderful energy. We must honor that the very system of Reiki was born through the curiosity and spiritual quest of a man who believed there was more to life and healing than what he knew or had been told. The energy of Reiki has many secrets to reveal to us. If we remain content that those before us knew all that there is to know, we will never move forward into the promise of what Reiki is capable of offering: not only a transformation of individuals but a transformation of all humanity as well.

2

Attunements and Degrees

There are three degrees in Reiki. In First Degree Reiki, the energy flows out of your hands. In Second Degree, you learn Reiki symbols for empowering the flow of Reiki, so you can send it across time and space, or direct it to heal mental and emotional issues. Third Degree Reiki is the Master Level, where you are empowered with more symbols, which allows you to perform the sacred attunement ceremony. Some teachers break the Third Degree up into two levels, teaching Reiki as a Four Degree system, offering the energetic empowerment of Master Level as the Third Degree to students who want to flow higher levels of energy but who do not want to go on to become Reiki Masters. In that system, they then treat the Fourth Degree as the final Master Level training.

The Attunement Initiation

Learning Reiki is something that requires an initiation, called an attunement. You cannot access Reiki simply through intellectual or meditative means. There are attunements for each level of Reiki that open the hands and crown chakra to the energy of Reiki at each level. (For those unfamiliar with the term, chakras are sacred energy wheels that exist at seven places in our energetic body, starting at the bottom of the torso and moving upward. The crown chakra, which is at the very top of the skullcap, both influences and is influenced by our spiritual awareness and connection to the Divine.) Traditionally these attunements are performed in person by a Reiki Master. The unique thing about this book is that it reveals a new method of attunement that allows easy access for all to be attuned to Reiki without going to a Reiki Master. The intention of this is to provide all of humanity with the capacity to use Reiki in their lives every day for health and spiritual growth. It is not the intent of this book to certify or train people as Reiki practitioners working on a professional level. If you want to become a Reiki practitioner and use Reiki professionally, the best thing would be to go to a Reiki Master and become trained, with individual attention suited to your questions and needs.

Reiki for All

Unfortunately, as a species in spiritual and ecological crisis, we do not have the time or resources for everyone to be individually trained in Reiki. Economics gets in the way, as does the suspicion of many who do not want to invest large sums of time, energy, and money in a method of healing that is generally based on something invisible. It is important, then, to provide Reiki to humanity in a way that is useful, easy, and accessible. And all humans do need Reiki, for their own health, for the sake of elevating the entire vibration of the human race, and for the sake of the planet as a whole.

There are some in the old school of Reiki who would say that Reiki does not belong to all people, that it is reserved for the spiritually evolved. They would say as well that it is a power that must be earned and not given away. To a certain point, I agree with the argument that it is not to be given away. I have attuned a few people for free who did not seem to appreciate their new capacity to heal. Reiki is a sacred energy, and there are some who will not recognize it as such. There are some who will take this gift for granted and not fully recognize the power that it can bring into their lives. But we cannot hold back on offering Reiki to all of humanity because of these individuals. And the current test for becoming a Reiki practitioner is unfortunately mostly financial. There seems to be very little spirituality in that measure. So I offer this book to those who want to get their feet wet in the Reiki System of Natural Healing. I also offer it to those who wish to discover the infinite capacity for Reiki to influence their lives. The concept of an energy exchange is not ignored in this book, but it has been shifted to try and make Reiki available to everyone.

Expanding the Attunement Process

After studying the sacred symbols used in the Reiki system, and after several years of experimenting with them and teaching them to others, I have discovered that there are a variety of attunement techniques and possibilities. First, it is possible to send a Reiki attunement across time and space. Essentially that means that any Reiki Master can initiate anyone on the planet at any point in time—in the past, present, or future. That might be a little hard to swallow, but it is the truth. Second, one Reiki attunement can initiate multiple individuals to Reiki, as long as the attunement is sent directly to that group of individuals. Third, a Reiki attunement can be activated via an action, statement, or any act of will that places an individual, or group of individuals, in the path of the intent of the attunement.

These three principles are not commonly known in the world of Reiki, and have only been discovered through years of intensive experimentation. This new method of attuning people to Reiki should not be discounted just because our teachers did not know about it. I have experimented for over a decade in using this method with consenting individuals who were not previously attuned to Reiki. Each time it has proven effective and demonstrates the capacity for efficiently expanding the circle of Reiki light to all of humanity.

Using the three principles that I have outlined above, let us now move forward into the realm of initiation into Reiki. But please read all of chapter 3 before using the chant that is offered for one to become attuned. It is important to understand the consequences of accepting a Reiki attunement, and to agree to the energy exchange involved.

3
First Degree Reiki Initiation

I have sent a Reiki attunement across all time and space to all individuals who say the Reiki First Degree Attunement Chant revealed later in this chapter. At that time, I will also offer more specific instructions and suggestions for using the chant. If you say this chant with the intent of being attuned to the First Degree of Reiki, you will be attuned in the act of saying the phrase. This works because the attunement has been sent out across time and space to intersect with anyone who says the Reiki First Degree Attunement Chant while intending to be attuned.

What you should know before asking for this is that the attunement will change your overall vibration, raising it to a higher level. For some people, this is a wonderful experience. For everyone, it is a healing experience. But for a few people, the healing experience can mean shedding old emotional walls that have repressed wounds from the past. At times, an attunement will lead to radical changes in how we eat, think, work, and whom we relate to. If you are not ready to embrace such possible change, it may not be wise at this time to go forward with the attunement.

Energy Exchange for Attunement

Traditionally Reiki requires some form of energy exchange to become attuned. Though I do believe in the energy exchange, I do not believe that it always needs to be monetary. I also do not believe that it needs to be directly given to the Reiki Master. The attunement comes from the Divine, and what is important is an act of gratitude for this gift. Generally the act of gratitude would be toward the Reiki Master, who has taken time and energy to perform the sacred attunement process. This concept has become warped at times, leading some people to pay huge sums of money for the right to be blessed with Reiki. Though huge sums of money are not necessary, I do agree that something should be given back.

Since I am not taking away from my personal time to attune each and every one who says the Attunement Chant, I do not feel it is right for me to ask for anything other than what I might make as the author of this book. But I do think that it is important for each individual to make a commitment before asking for the attunement. Commit to do some act of good works, or to give money to a charity. Why not use your newfound gift of Reiki to help bring healing to people in a nursing home, or to help an animal or plant that is suffering? I suggest that the best way for you to extend the circle of healing light and also to show the Divine that you are thankful for this new gift is to give three hours of Reiki without thought or request for compensation. Meditate on what you plan to do to complete the energy exchange.

Preparation for Attunement

When you are ready, set a date when you want to receive the First Degree Reiki attunement. You might wish to align this special day with an important day on your own spiritual calendar, or in keeping with the phases of the moon or the seasons. In any case, set aside the whole day for this occasion.

On the day you have chosen for the attunement, take a long sea-salt bath in the morning. This will help relax you and also clean your aura. After your bath, get into some comfortable clothing, something loose and relaxing to wear. Then go into a quiet room, or to a place in nature that feels special or sacred. If you have an altar for your own spiritual practice, you might wish to sit in front of the altar. Let your inner self guide you to the best place to receive your sacred attunement.

Though it is not required, I suggest lighting a white candle in honor of Dr. Usui for returning the gift of Reiki to humanity at this time in our evolution. Though he did not invent Reiki and is not the source of Reiki, it was through his spiritual search that Reiki was returned to humanity. (My own spirit guides say that humanity has had the capacity for Reiki at various times, in Atlantis and in Egypt and perhaps elsewhere. The problem is that human ego and arrogance has always gotten in the way, resulting in spiritual aristocracies where some people were forbidden the light in order to keep others in a position of power and control. Let us make sure that we learn our karmic lesson as a whole and allow the light to spread to all this time.)

Besides lighting a candle to Dr. Usui, I also suggest you light a candle to the Divine, in whatever form you see it. Reiki does come from the Divine, and since this ritual is for you, there is no harm in expressing your gratitude personally.

The Attunement Experience

Having lit your candles and entered your sacred space for this attunement, allow yourself to quiet your mind. And when the spirit moves you, repeat the chant:

> *Blessed be the Ones who brought us Reiki*
> *Blessed be the Ones who continue this sacred light*
> *I ask for the attunement of Reiki First Degree*
> *Blessings unto all*
> *Blessings unto me*

It is necessary to say the chant only once. But if you feel inspired, you can say it as many times as you wish. In saying the chant, you intersect with the attunement that has been sent out to all who say this chant with the intent of becoming attuned. Though some might argue against the accuracy of such an attunement method, it has been tested numerous times since I began experimenting with it in 1995 and it has never failed. Also, all Reiki Masters know that the only difference between First and Second Degree attunements is the intention of the Reiki Master. All Reiki Masters know as well the power of certain symbols in Reiki to transcend time and space. Hence, the concept of intention and the concept of transcending time and space are already inherent in Reiki. All that is happening with this attunement method is that those concepts are joined together using a chant as the vehicle to help target the attunement to the appropriate people.

Once attuned to First Degree Reiki, you might wish to take some time to just be with yourself. Often the precious minutes after an attunement can be very special. Depending of how sensitive you are to subtle energy, you may or may not feel the difference immediately in your head or your hands. Try to realize that there is no one right way to experience the attunement. If the changes feel minimal, or unnoticeable, do not fear. You have been attuned, and the energy of Reiki will flow through your hands now.

Once the attunement happens, it is important to know that the energy flowing through your hands will grow stronger the more you use it. When I was attuned to First Degree Reiki, I hardly noticed any shift in the energy coming out of my hands even though I was already a psychic and energy healer. But over time, the vibration became stronger. Some people have "hot hands" and will notice the shift immediately. Know that whatever you feel is right for you. Treat this day as sacred, and know that your vibration has now been changed for life, raised to a higher level.

Traditionally teaching was given immediately after the attunement on how to use Reiki for yourself and how to give a Reiki treatment to another person. But since you have this book and can go at your own pace, you may wish to take your time to celebrate this sacred occasion. Or, if you prefer, you may wish to follow tradition and go immediately into using Reiki on yourself. Do whatever feels right to you, and let your own intuition be your guide.

4

The Reiki Self-Treatment

Once you have been attuned to Reiki, the first thing you need to learn is how to use this sacred energy system for healing yourself. The Reiki self-treatment is very simple, and can be used whenever you need it. I strongly suggest that you use it at least once a day for the twenty-one days following the attunement. During this twenty-one-day period, major shifts usually occur because of the change in your energy vibration. Your body might be releasing toxins, old emotional memories, or adjusting to new conditions that have been caused by the raised vibration. It is important to help your body through this time by giving yourself Reiki. I also suggest drinking lots of water during this time, as this helps the kidneys release toxins that the body is now ready to shed.

The Self-Treatment Process

To begin the Reiki self-treatment, you should lie down comfortably on a bed or on the floor. It can be done sitting in a chair as well, but most people prefer lying down. Wash your hands so they are clean. The washing represents entering the space of the Reiki treatment with a clear and pure intention. It also helps prevent contaminating the eyes, since the eyes are the first part of the body treated.

Eyes

Place the palms of your hands gently over your eyes, allowing them to rest and without applying pressure. Your fingers should be together, not splayed. You do not need to do anything to make the Reiki flow, and should think of it as a Divine river that you cannot push. It will simply flow, and all you need to do is allow it. Again, you may not feel anything at first. Most people will have a tingling or warm sensation moving out of their hands, but not everyone will experience this. So do not worry if you do not feel anything. Simply allow the Reiki to do what it needs to do, remembering that it is being directed by the Divine and has an intelligent nature. Hold this position for three to five minutes.

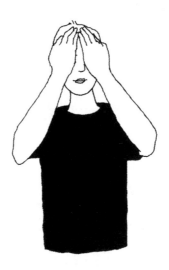

You may notice that your breathing changes during this time. I often experience a deep sigh when going into the first few minutes of a Reiki treatment. You may feel calm or settled, maybe even sleepy. Remember that this process is moving through you, and it is not your energy but the Divine's energy that is causing the healing. Simply let go and just be, even if that means you do not feel anything. The important thing is to stick with it, keeping your hands in the same position.

Head

Once the eyes are treated for several minutes, slide your hands to the side of your head so that your palms are now resting over each temple. Keep your hands there for another three- to five-minute period. Over time, you will eventually come to sense the right time to move from one position to another. You will be able to listen to information that comes to you through your hands. But for now, use the three- to five-minute period for each position.

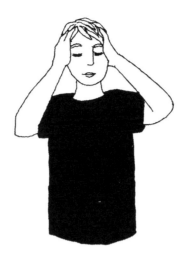

When you have finished treating the temples, slide your hands so that your palms are now covering your ears. Just let your hands rest, while letting the Reiki flow for three to five minutes.

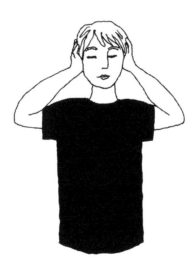

After working on your ears, slide your hands along your jaws. This is an excellent area to work on if you have problems with temporo-mandibular joint (TMJ) disorder or difficulty expressing anger. Many times we can store our feelings of anger in our jaws, and Reiki can be very useful in releasing tension from this part of our bodies. Hold this position for the same amount of time as the other positions.

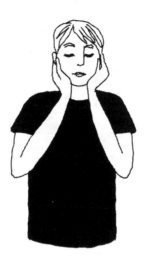

Front Sides of Torso

Next, start a series of positions that are like two stripes, one down each side of the front of your torso, by bringing your hands to each side of your upper chest, fingertips resting on the collarbone halfway between

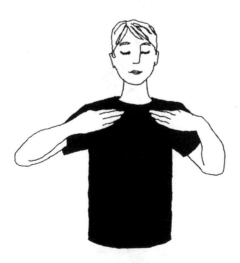

your shoulder and neck on the left and right sides of your body. Adjust to your own comfort zone with this position. If anything feels like a stretch, or in any way uncomfortable, shift your hands so that you are not stressing yourself. This is not yoga, and we must allow our physical differences to speak and then listen to what is said. What works well for me may not be exactly what you need. So see these positions as approximations, not fixed targets. The Reiki has intelligence and will flow where it needs to go.

After working the upper chest, slide your hands down covering each breast, essentially performing Reiki on the lungs and surrounding muscle tissue. Your fingers should still be together, not splayed. As with the other positions, keep your hands in this place for three to five minutes. Working the lungs is important. I have often found that five minutes of Reiki can end congestion when I feel the first symptoms of a chest cold coming on.

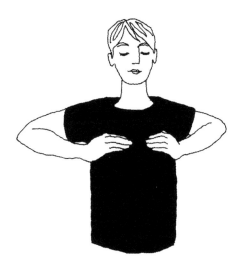

The next position is the lower rib cage. Again, slide your hands gently. Keep your hands slightly to the side, as later you will come back and work down the front and middle of the body.

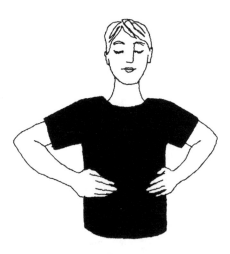

From this point, after the period of appropriate time, slide your hands down to the sides of your abdomen. Treat this area for three to five minutes.

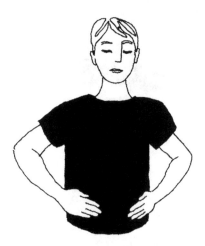

For the last position of this series, though not the entire session, place your hands so that your palms are resting on your waist, over your hip sockets. Hold this position for three to five minutes. You have now finished the two stripes down the sides of your torso.

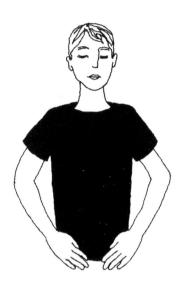

Center of Torso

Return to the neck, and now work a series of positions that cover the center of the torso. Begin with your palms hovering just above your throat, an inch or two away from your Adam's apple. This area tends to be very sensitive, and does not need to be touched. The Reiki will flow from your palms to your throat. Direct contact is not necessary. (In actuality, direct contact is never entirely necessary. I have known a few Reiki practitioners who do not touch any position during a Reiki treatment. I prefer direct contact when possible, as do most Reiki practitioners. Most people like to feel the warmth of a hand that is flowing Reiki. But if you prefer to hover your hands in each position instead of making direct contact, that will also work.) Hold this position for three to five minutes. This area is extremely important for those who need to work on expressing themselves emotionally. This position covers the throat chakra, the energy center that governs human communication. I have found that a good dose of Reiki in this position is very effective in clearing a sore throat, and in mending relationships and friendships where one person is not speaking out.

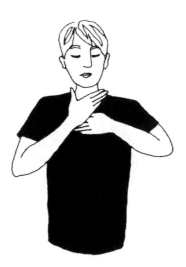

After working the throat, slide your hands down so that they are adjacent to each other, palms covering the region of the heart chakra, not the physical heart. The heart chakra is located in the center of the chest, a few inches above the diaphragm. This is a great area to work for helping

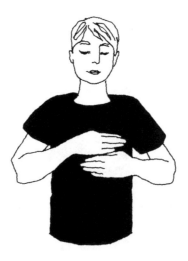

clear up issues of the heart, and Reiki will flow to the physical heart from this position as well. Hold this position for three to five minutes.

Next, slide your hands down so that they are still adjacent to each other, covering the region between the navel and the diaphragm. This covers the region of your power chakra, and helps restore a sense of will and empowerment. It also aids in digestion. Hold this position for three to five minutes.

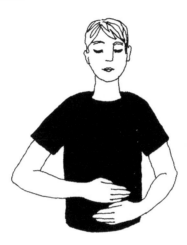

For the next position, slide your hands down so that the region between the navel and the upper pelvis is covered. Here Reiki flows into the chakra governing sexuality, aiding the creative flow of a person. Hold this position for three to five minutes.

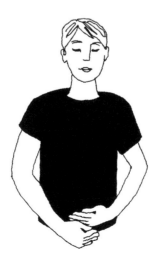

The final position of this series, though not of the whole session, involves making a "T" by hovering the left hand over the genitals with the fingers pointing horizontally toward the right hip, meanwhile holding the right hand so that the right wrist is touching the left hand and the right fingers are pointing down toward the anus. This covers both the sex organs and root chakra, the most primal regions of our being. Hold this position for three to five minutes.

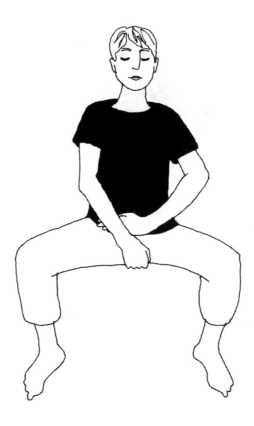

Back of Head and Torso

Now, it is time to perform Reiki on the back of the head. Place both hands behind your head, in any manner that is comfortable. Hold this position for three to five minutes.

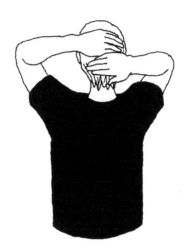

After treating the back of the head, bring your hands down to your back just below the rib cage. Reiki here will reach the kidneys, and help flush out toxins released by the attunement and the self-treatment session. Hold this position for three to five minutes.

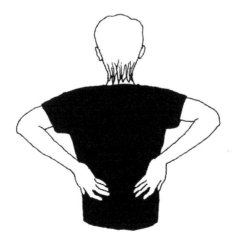

Next, slide your hands so that they are covering your coccyx, or tailbone. Hold this position for three to five minutes, or longer if you are prone to lower back problems.

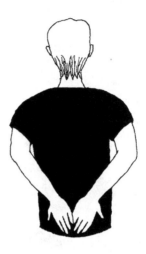

Knees and Feet

The knees are the next position. Place one hand on each knee, and let the Reiki flow for three to five minutes.

The final position involves grabbing the arches of your feet. Let the Reiki flow into this region, which helps ground you and return you to a centered place for the end of the treatment. Hold this position for three to five minutes.

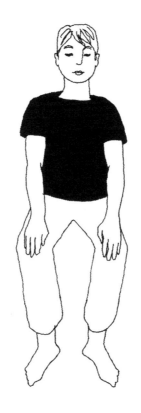

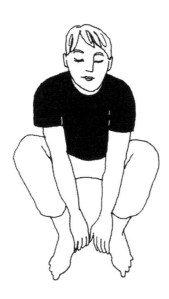

After the Self-Treatment

When you have finished a Reiki self-treatment, thank the energy and beings that have brought this healing to you. I use the term "Beings of Reiki" to include any Reiki Masters from the past who helped bring the gift of Reiki to me. It also might include angels, Devas, or other spirit beings who have aided me in having this capacity to perform Reiki. Naturally I consider the Divine to be a Being of Reiki as well. I simply say, "I thank the Beings of Reiki for this gift of healing." The last thing I do after each session is wash my hands. This has the symbolic message of cleansing and releasing. It serves a physical function of cleaning the hands as well.

One important note is that you do not always have to do a full self-treatment to experience Reiki. You can always just place your hand on any area of your body that seems to need Reiki at any time and allow the flow to occur. This is especially true when you are ill or injured. The self-treatment should be done regularly, once a day. But do not limit yourself to only doing Reiki on yourself in this self-treatment sequence. For more daily uses of Reiki, see the following chapter.

5

Daily Uses of Reiki

Reiki is more than just a tool for self-healing. It as an energy that can connect us more deeply with the Divine, as well with all beings with which we interact. It can even enhance the nutrients we put into our own bodies. One Reiki Master who taught me used the analogy of Reiki being like a sacred dye: each time we dip the fabric of our being into it, our own sacred nature further reveals itself. In keeping with her analogy, below are a few brief suggestions about how to dip even further into Reiki on a daily basis.

Reiki Treatments of Food

One extension of performing Reiki treatments on yourself is to perform them on all that you eat. Food provides us not only with nutrients, but the vibrations of the food become part of us as well. If your food vibrates from a place of love and light, then naturally it will be more beneficial to you. I perform Reiki on my food by simply holding my hands a few inches above a meal before I eat it. The Reiki will flow into the food just as it flows into your throat when holding your palms a few inches away from your throat during a treatment. Reiki will also go through a cup or glass into any drinks that you wish to treat with Reiki before consuming. I cannot say that the taste actually changes, but the food does possess a certain quality when treated with Reiki. This quality is something tangible, which affects all that you are since the food is literally becoming part of you. Some Reiki Masters recommend long treatments of certain foods before eating to help in purifying the body of toxins and disease.

Reiki for Plants, Animals, and Inanimate Objects

You can also give Reiki to plants, animals, and inanimate objects. I often give Reiki to trees when I am walking, especially in a town or city where trees are cut off from forests or large natural areas. After some time, you can become sensitive to the fact that trees growing in a small patch of dirt near a sidewalk often have a fairly weak life force when compared to the energy of a tree in the woods. Trees, houseplants, and garden flowers can all use Reiki. And in giving Reiki, the Reiki flows through you so that you are also receiving it.

Animals are usually receptive to Reiki as well. I have done Reiki on several dogs, which have fallen asleep during a treatment. I just put my hands where the animal will allow and let the Reiki flow. There have been a few times when the animal did not seem to understand what is happening. If an animal gets startled or confused, end the treatment immediately. Whatever healing you might be bringing to the animal will be offset by the confusion they are experiencing.

Inanimate objects can be treated with Reiki to improve their functional capacity. I have heard stories of people starting dead car batteries with Reiki. And though I cannot say I have experienced that personally, I have helped start a few lawn mowers with a short treatment of Reiki to a machine that was not working only minutes before. How this works exactly, I cannot say. Perhaps when PhDs in nuclear physics and electrical engineering become Reiki Masters, we will have a greater understanding of this dynamic. My guess is that the changes that occur on a molecular level during a Reiki treatment are enough, in some cases, to shift and release some electrical problems. Reiki is not going to fix a broken window or inflate a flat tire. But using Reiki on appliances can apparently aid in their functioning, and also serves to keep you using and flowing with this wonderful gift.

6

Reiki Treatments for
Family and Friends

I want to emphasize that this book carries the power to attune you to Reiki, and my focus here is to bring Reiki into our daily lives. As I said earlier, if you wish to engage Reiki professionally, get professional training. There is no substitute for one-on-one attention to your technique and answers to the questions you are bound to have when pursuing the path of becoming a Reiki practitioner. Reading this book and asking for the attunements to be given does not qualify you to charge money for your services any more than doing exercises from a book on massage qualifies you to be a massage therapist.

The flip side of this issue is that we must return to a greater sense of community if humanity is going to thrive or even survive. Using Reiki to help those close to you maintain health is encouraged. I hope that the following treatment will foster a sense of people taking care of each other, and that it will not be used to promote financial gain by the untrained practitioner.

The untrained practitioner must be warned as well that to accept this gift from the Divine with the manipulative intent of pretending to be a fully trained Reiki practitioner carries the weight of severe negative karma. You cannot benefit from such an action, and my warning should not be dismissed. The few times that I have seen people engage in any kind of deceptive act involving the acceptance of a Reiki attunement, the consequences have been severe. The One you would attempt to cheat is the All-Seeing and All-Powerful. Do not take this warning lightly.

Thus, you should be a friend or relative of the person you are working on. If the person being treated is ill or suffering from a specific condition, you will probably be aware of this. However, it is still wise to ask if there is anything specific that the person wishes to gain from the healing. Your grandmother might be suffering pain in her neck, but you may discover in talking to her that she wants the session to be more about helping her overcome the nagging influence of a particular family member. In any case, ask, listen, and let the Reiki respond.

I have found that Reiki is truly intelligent, and that the verbalized issue will always be addressed in some manner during a treatment. It may not entirely heal the issue, but it will open the path for that healing to move forward.

Preparation for the Treatment

The location where the treatment is performed is highly important: a quiet, peaceful setting where the person receiving the treatment can comfortably lie down is best. In the best scenario, you would use a massage table in a quiet, softly lit room that offered an ambience of serenity. But not everyone has this luxury, so use your best judgment in deciding which space to use for the treatment.

The person being treated should wear comfortable clothes, and lie down on a bed or on a mat on the floor. As I said above, Reiki is best done on a massage table, but as this is not a professional session, it is unlikely that most families will have one at their disposal. The person being treated should be on their back initially, with their arms and legs uncrossed. Ask the person to remove glasses, shoes, watches, and any jewelry. Hopefully, you will have a pillow and blanket available. The pillow, naturally, will rest under the person's head. The blanket should cover their feet, as you do not want their feet to get cold.

As with sessions on yourself, wash your hands to symbolize entering a clean and pure space of intention, as well as to keep from contaminating the person's eyes during the first position.

The Treatment Process

Reiki treatment is a sacred process during which the healer acts as a vessel for Divine Energy that flows through him or her into the person being healed. Reiki is both simple and Divine. It is important to remember that the energy is coming through you, not from you. In performing a Reiki treatment, you are also receiving Reiki yourself.

Prayer

Begin the session with a short prayer, asking that the session be for the highest good of all. I usually speak this from my heart, not out loud.

Sweep the Aura

Once you have said your prayer, begin by sweeping the aura with your hands very slowly from head to toe, making sure that you do not go from toe to head. The purpose of this is to smooth the aura, which has a very calming effect on most people. Going in the opposite direction actually ruffles the aura.

To sweep the aura, simply hold out your hands a few inches away from the person's physical body, palms facing down. You may want to pretend that the person is like a large cat, with invisible fur sticking out about six inches or more from the physical body. Though the aura is much further out than this, I find that six inches is a good measure for this technique. Using the image of a large cat, simply pretend you are petting this imaginary fur, and smoothing out any tangles. Over time, you will become sensitive to clogs in the energy field, just as you might notice clumps of fur when petting a cat. The analogy is fairly close. The more you pet those clumped areas, the more they become smooth.

I usually use three long slow strokes across the aura from head to toe. When I get to the feet, I pull my hands back away from the person's aura so that I do not ruffle it when going back up to their head. Smooth the aura three times, making sure each time that you are going gently and slowly. Fast sweeps across the aura can feel very startling and uncomfortable to people, especially those who are highly energy sensitive.

Eyes

Once you have smoothed the aura, place your hands lightly with your palms covering the person's eyes. You should do this from behind their head, so that your fingers are pointing down toward their chin, thumbs resting near the person's nose. Avoid putting any pressure on the nose or blocking the person's ability to breathe. Let the Reiki flow from your hands for three to five minutes. You do not need to visualize anything, or do anything to push this Divine river of energy. Your mind will often become very calm as the Reiki must flow through you to get to the person you are working on. Simply be in the space of allowing the Divine to do this healing through you. Nothing else is required.

Head

Once you have treated the eyes for the required time, slide your hands gently so that your palms are now covering the person's temples. Allow Reiki to flow through your hands for three to five minutes here. Remember, just as when you are doing a self-treatment, your fingers should be together, not splayed.

When working on a person's head, I will sometimes sense something about which they are thinking, perhaps issues or troubles that concern them. Being attuned to Reiki does not make you a professional counselor. If you do sense the person's thoughts, I simply suggest letting these impressions move through you with the Reiki. If a strong image keeps coming up and you have a very strong sense that it is information the person needs to have brought to light, then wait until the session is over and ask if the person would like to hear about any impressions you received during the session. They might say no, since what they have agreed to is a Reiki session and not a psychic reading. If the person does say no, always respect his or her wishes. It is part of the holy healing space you are entering to respect the freewill choice of the person on whom you are working. But if he or she says yes, convey your impressions in a way that is gentle and respectful of the boundaries of that person.

After treating the person's temples, slide your hands so that your palms are covering their ears. Hold this position for three to five minutes.

Once the ears have been treated, slide your hands so that your fingers are along the person's jaw on each side, pointing toward their chin. Your palms should be near the person's jaw hinge on each side. Again, just as in a self-treatment, this is an excellent area to work on for a person who holds in unexpressed anger or physical tension.

Once you have treated the jaws fully for three to five minutes, turn the person's head slightly to one side so that you may slip one hand under their head. Then gently turn the person's head to the other side and slip your other hand under their head as well. The person's skull is now resting in your palms, with Reiki flowing directly into the back of their brain.

I have found most people thoroughly enjoy having this area worked on. Often people who seem to be fighting the flow of Reiki into their bodies will surrender at this point and allow themselves to really let the Reiki come in. You might hear them give a deep sigh, if they haven't already done so. Their breathing will relax into a much deeper and calm rhythm. These things often happen earlier in the session, but occasionally some people resist allowing the Reiki to flow into them. For whatever reason, they have difficulty allowing themselves to receive.

Occasionally you may treat people who, on some level, do not really want Reiki. You may feel your hands are very hot, and that the Reiki is flowing through you very strongly, but nothing seems to happen to the person being treated. The person's breathing does not deepen, nor does he or she seem to relax. If this happens, just know that the person has chosen on some level not to allow the Reiki to come in. Reiki will not violate free will and will not enter if the person does not really want it. There is no need for blame or guilt when this happens. Just realize it is part of the person's freewill choice, and that you have done your part by offering your hands in service of the Divine. Do not blame the person for making this choice, as it is probably being made on a subconscious level. Simply allow the person the space to have his or her own experience and reaction, knowing you have done your best.

Shoulders

After treating the back of the head for three to five minutes, gently slide your hands out from beneath the person's skull and place them on the person's shoulders. Acupuncture meridians travel from the shoulders all the way down to the legs and feet. This is one of the positions where Reiki will often be felt through the whole body by the person who is receiving the treatment, as the energy will often move like a flowing river through those meridians. Hold this position for the three- to five-minute period, keeping your fingers together and making sure that you are comfortable in how your own body is positioned.

People can sense it if you are stressing your body or uncomfortable in giving a Reiki treatment. Your comfort is not something that is to be ignored when giving Reiki. Though I prefer standing when working next to a table or bed, and crouching down when on the floor, some people prefer using a chair, pillows, or whatever is necessary to keep themselves comfortable. This makes the session an experience that is pleasurable for both parties. Use your own common sense to determine what you need to do to maintain your personal comfort, as long as it is not at the expense of the person you are working on. Lying next to someone or invading their personal space is not the appropriate solution. Be aware of both your needs and the needs of the person you are treating, and use common sense.

Torso Front

Once you have fully treated the person's shoulders, it is time to decide which side you want to be on when treating the rest of the body. Move from behind the head to either the left or right side of the torso. It does not matter which side, as long as you and the person you are working on are comfortable.

Now, place one hand at the top of the sternum, just below the person's neck. Lay this hand flat, and rest your other hand at a forty-five-degree angle on top of it so that it is slanted several inches away from the throat. This allows you to hold your hand near the person's throat without directly touching it. As with the Reiki self-treatment, you want to avoid direct contact with the throat, which is highly sensitive. Allow Reiki to flow here for three to five minutes.

For the next position, if you are working on a man place your hands over the center of the person's chest, letting Reiki flow into the heart and lungs. If you are working on a woman, you may prefer to keep the one hand on the sternum and place the other hand on top of it at a forty-five-degree angle in the direction of the woman's chest, so that the fingers are pointing down toward her legs, hovering over her heart but not touching. Essentially, you are performing the same "T" formation over her breasts that you used when treating your genitals and root chakra during the Reiki self-treatment. Depending on the comfort zone between the two of you, this alternative position may or may not be necessary. If the comfort zone is in question, use the "T" formation.

After working on the heart and chest, gently move your hands to the lower rib cage on each side of the person. Allow Reiki to flow here for three to five minutes.

Now, move your hands so that they are covering the abdomen above the navel. Treat this area for the three- to five-minute time frame. When you are finished working above the navel, slide your hands so that they are covering the abdomen between the navel and pelvis. Allow Reiki to flow here for another three- to five-minute period.

Coming to the pelvis, I prefer to put my hands to the sides of the hips and let the Reiki flow through my hands across the pelvis entirely. Reiki will flow very strong between your hands across the pelvis. Thus using this technique allows a full treatment of the pelvis without encroaching on anyone's sexual boundaries. Treat for the usual three- to five-minute period.

Knees and Feet

Next, come down to the knees and put one hand on each knee. Allow Reiki to flow here for the usual time. If someone seems to be suffering from knee trouble, I will treat each knee individually with both hands, placing one hand above the knee and one hand below. In such cases I treat each knee for three to five minutes. But normally, you can treat both knees simultaneously for the usual three- to five-minute period.

When finishing treating the knees, come down to the person's feet and grab each arch, allowing the curve of your hand to embrace the curve of their arch in each foot. Hold this position for three to five minutes, and then gently ask the person to slowly roll over and face downward.

Torso Back

Once the person is facing down, come up and treat the back of the shoulder blades. This position also flows Reiki again to the lungs. Hold this position for the three- to five-minute time period.

The back of the heart chakra is perhaps the best region to treat for someone going through sadness or grief, or who simply needs to cry.

Often people will try to hold in their feelings when facing you during the treatment. But when they face down, their eyes are shielded from you and most people seem more able to let go at this point. Treat the back of the heart chakra after working on the shoulder blades. Simply hold both hands in the center of the back between the shoulder blades. The treatment should go for the usual three to five minutes, unless the person is experiencing the kind of emotional release mentioned above. In such cases, I recommend holding the position long enough to allow the person to move fully through the emotional release.

When you have finished working on the back of the heart chakra, slide your hands down to just beneath the bottom of the rib cage. This area will allow Reiki to flow directly to the kidneys. Treat this area for three to five minutes.

Next is the only position that does not have a general time frame. It is called "balancing the spine" and requires putting one hand on the tailbone and the other at the C-7 vertebra where the neck is joined to the torso. Let Reiki flow through your hands, and you will notice that one hand will feel hotter or more vibrant than the other. Hold this position until both hands feel the same amount of heat or vibration. When your hands have come into harmony in this manner, it means that the energy of the spine is balanced.

Back of Knees and Feet

The next position is the back of the knees. Treat this area for three to five minutes, even if you have treated each knee individually previously.

The final position involves returning to the feet and again matching the curve of your hand into the arch of each foot. Hold this position for the full five minutes to allow the person time to ground his or her energy.

Sweep the Aura Again

Finish the session by again sweeping the aura three times, using slow and gentle sweeps. After the third sweep, pull your hands together as though getting ready to say a prayer, and point your fingertips down toward the spine at the bottom of the person's tailbone, not actually touching him or her but several inches away. Imagine a red laser beam of light coming out of your fingertips and into the person's spine.

Moving slowly, keep your hand floating above the spine and move toward the skull, imagining the red laser beam of light still coming out of your hands into the spine. As you walk this red light up the spine, you help revitalize the person's energy and bring him or her closer to a state of normal waking consciousness.

Thanksgiving and Conclusion Session

When you get to the bottom of the skull, point your fingertips up toward the sky and mentally thank the person for allowing you to perform this treatment. Also mentally thank yourself for being part of this process. And finish with thanks to the Divine and all Beings of Reiki. Then wipe your hands together, to signify that the treatment is done. Quietly tell the person to get up when ready. Then go wash your hands.

After washing your hands you may want to check in with the person you have just treated. See how the person is and offer a glass of juice or water. Remember, a full session of Reiki can leave people feeling so wonderfully relaxed that they might not think to take care of themselves. But getting fluids into the body after a session helps the body flush toxins that are released by the treatment. The full impact of the treatment might last for as long as three days, so encourage the person you treated to drink lots of fluids during that time.

Intuitive Treatment

The above treatment is a guide, not a steadfast rule. You should probably stay true to it until you come to trust and listen to your hands. Eventually your hands will know where to go. You will intuitively know where to put them during a session, which might also mean holding some positions for long periods of time or finding positions not mentioned in the treatment above. Listening to your hands is something that takes practice.

Though not included in the traditional hand positions, I have often found myself called to give Reiki to a person's elbow or arm, only to later discover that the person had recently suffered an injury in that area. Reiki is intelligent, and will communicate to you through your hands and perhaps other senses as well. However, this takes time as well as a willingness to trust and listen, but the effort is worth it. At times I have even received audible messages that suggest changes in diet or attitude for the person I am working on. When I share those messages, they always seem to resonate very clearly with the person.

There is a difference between getting messages and hearing a person's thoughts. A person's thoughts are theirs, and not a place for me to tread unless invited to share what I picked up. Messages, however, are something I feel obligated to share.

In the beginning, however, you should simply concentrate on doing a thorough treatment, making sure that all the positions have been treated for the three- to five-minute period.

Just as with the Reiki self-treatment, realize that it is okay to give a person a limited treatment to a specific area. You do not always have to give a full-body treatment, especially if there are restrictions of time. If someone has a stomachache and needs a ten-minute session on the stomach to help him or her through the day, then place your hands on the stomach. Do not feel compelled to give a full-body treatment every time you use Reiki. A full-body Reiki treatment is ideal but not always possible.

7

Group Treatments

Group Reiki can be one of the most pleasurable aspects of Reiki. As more hands are put on one person, the Reiki seems to be amplified exponentially. When treating someone in a group session, you can often get the same amount of healing in ten minutes that would normally take an entire session. There are pitfalls, however. These occur most often when the competitive egos of the people performing Reiki get in the way. Sometimes one person might want to "take control," turning the healing space into an ego space. Or, sometimes the hand positions are not in sequence because not everyone involved has had the same Reiki Master or been given the same teachings. This leads to a sense of confusion within the group that is very often felt by the person being worked on.

Coordinating a Group Treatment

The most effective means I have seen for avoiding problems within a group treatment is to decide beforehand exactly how long each treatment will be. Have one person smooth the aura. Then, depending on how many practicing Reiki hands are available, each person holds only one position while the person being treated is facing up. Even if there are only two Reiki people working on someone, having one person working on the eyes and the other on the feet sends enough Reiki through the whole body to be effective. Remember, the treatment is highly amplified as more hands are added. If a third is available, he or she can work on the abdomen. If more are available, you can have two people on the left and right sides of the body working on the heart chakra and power chakra simultaneously, while the other two are at the head and feet. Moving from one position to another simply is not necessary in a group treatment.

When treatment on the front side is finished, ask the person to turn over slowly. Then do a blanket treatment across the spine. This feels fabulous, and is perhaps the best experience I have ever had in Reiki. Simply have all the available Reiki hands lined up along the person's spine. Holding this position even for just a few minutes provides an incredible experience for the person who is receiving the treatment. When you are finished, have one person ground out the session by working on the feet, smoothing the aura, and adding the final wake-up call of red light to the spine.

By having no changes in the hand positions, and agreeing how long the session should be beforehand, issues about control and ego are less likely to arise.

Be simple, and a group treatment can be a true gift for everyone involved.

8

Second Degree Reiki Symbols

Three symbols are traditionally learned in Second Degree Reiki. These symbols are used to empower the flow of Reiki, invoke mental healing or protection, and send Reiki through the matrix of time/space. The capacity for changing one's life with these three symbols is immense.

Cho Ku Rei

The first symbol is the power symbol, which is called Cho Ku Rei. It is used to empower the flow of Reiki. When doing a hands-on treatment, it increases the heat or vibration of Reiki flowing through a person's hands. A diagram of the symbol is below. Each of the traditional Reiki

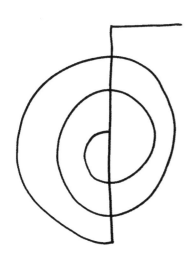

Cho Ku Rei

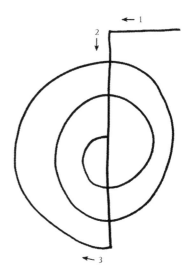

This is how the symbol is drawn

symbols is to be drawn in a particular fashion. Using a pen and paper, practice drawing Cho Ku Rei as shown by the numbers and arrows in the diagram on the right.

I recommend filling up one or two sheets of paper with the symbol. You cannot access the power of this symbol until you are attuned to Second Degree Reiki, but knowing how to draw it helps you internalize the image so you can visualize it during treatments after you are attuned to Second Degree Reiki. Visualizing the symbol, and chanting the name of the symbol either mentally or aloud, are the ways that the power of the symbol is accessed once you are attuned to Second Degree Reiki. If you are not sure how to pronounce it, here's how: Cho rhymes with Joe, Ku rhymes with Sue, and Rei rhymes with Jay.

For now, simply practice drawing the symbol and chanting the name. Later you will learn more about using it.

Sei He Ki

The second Reiki symbol is called Sei He Ki and pronounced "say hay key." This symbol is used for mental and emotional healing, and can be used also for protection. In both cases, it needs to be empowered by the Cho Ku Rei symbol in order to be effective. How this is done will be

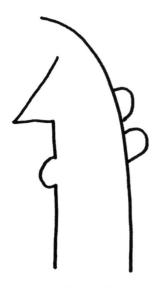

Sei He Ki

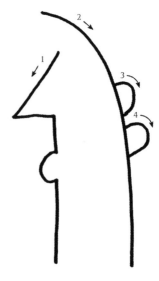

This is how the symbol is drawn

described later. But remember that, used by itself, it is like a flashlight with no battery. You must use this symbol in conjunction with Cho Ku Rei in order for it to have power. However, once empowered, Sei He Ki can be used to untangle the deepest emotional wounds and enlighten one as to the true nature of emotional entanglements. I have used it when no psychic or shamanic technique would help me, and have found it to be the one true remedy that I trust for all problems of the mind and heart. Just as with Cho Ku Rei, practice drawing and chanting this symbol.

Practice drawing the symbol as shown by the numbers and arrows.

Hon Sha Ze Sho Nen

The third symbol is the most mystical of the three. It is called Hon Sha Ze Sho Nen and allows one to send Reiki across all time, all space, and all dimensions. Here's the pronunciation: Hon rhymes with bone,

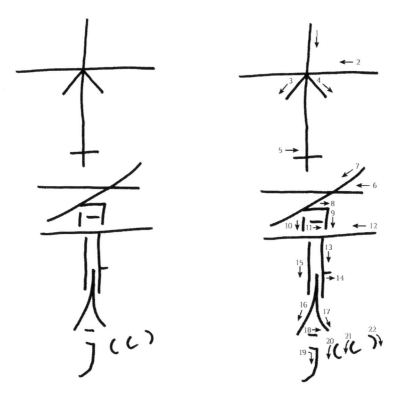

Hon Sha Ze Sho Nen   This is how the symbol is drawn

Sha rhymes with saw, Ze rhymes with jay, Sho rhymes with no, and Nen rhymes with Ben. It is much more complex to draw than the other two.

Practice chanting the name of the symbol and drawing it. This one will probably take you some time to memorize. Make sure you get each line in the right order and drawn in the right direction.

You should spend a day or two really learning the symbols before moving on to the Second Degree Reiki attunement. Once you have learned the symbols and go on to be attuned, you will have a profound way of empowering your life and of healing wounds from the past. The only real limit to your use of Second Degree Reiki is your imagination. As long as you honor the free will of other beings, your capacity to use these symbols is infinite. Techniques for their use and suggested exercises can be found in the following chapters.

9

Second Degree Reiki Attunement

The Second Degree Reiki Attunement is truly transformational, as it opens you to be able to offer healings through all time and space, something that can literally change how you think about the universe in which we live. Know that once you are attuned to Reiki at this level, your consciousness will be forever opened to the majestic fabric of the time/space matrix.

Energy Exchange for Attunement

Just as with the attunement in First Degree Reiki, you should make a commitment to do some act of good works or to give something to charity after you are attuned. The concept of energy exchange exists at all levels of the attunement process, and to abandon it is only to disregard the Divine and the great gift you are receiving with Reiki. This attunement is more powerful than the First Degree attunement, and it is strongly suggested that your energy exchange reflect a higher degree of commitment on your part. If you are happy with what you did for the First Degree Reiki attunement energy exchange, then I recommend you double that energy exchange in time, money, or effort.

You may wish to consider a commitment to send Reiki to the earth for healing our planet. Six hours of Reiki from one person may not change the world, but imagine what might happen if all the people who read this book committed to sending six hours of Reiki for planetary healing. Since Reiki has intelligence, sending Reiki to heal the earth has an effect in the overall consciousness of the planet, as well as the decisions made by governments, corporations, and individuals with respect to the planet. I can think of no better gift to give the earth than to use your new Reiki abilities to help the planet heal.

Preparation for Attunement

Once you have decided what your commitment will be, pick a date on which you would like to receive the attunement. Again, you may wish to pick a day that matches an important day on your own spiritual path, or you might pick a day more personally relevant like your birthday.

On the day of the attunement, take a sea-salt bath in the morning to clean your aura. Find a special or sacred space where you would like to receive the attunement. Again, this may be in nature or some other place that feels right to you. Just as before, I suggest that you light a candle to Dr. Mikao Usui to offer thanks for his spiritual quest that returned Reiki to humanity. Again, this is a suggestion and not a requirement. You may also wish to light a candle to the Divine. The candles are suggested for honoring how Reiki was returned to humanity, and have no effect on the outcome of the attunement.

The Attunement Experience

When you are ready to be attuned to Second Degree Reiki, say the following chant with the intention of being attuned:

Blessed be the Ones who have brought us Reiki
Blessed be the Ones who continue this sacred light
I ask for the attunement of Reiki Second Degree
Blessings unto all
Blessings unto me

Allow yourself the time and space to fully absorb and enjoy the preciousness of this moment. You can say the chant more than once, but once is all it takes. If you wish to celebrate this occasion, then do so with the highest blessings, knowing that the information on how to use this gift is waiting for you and that you are now attuned to Second Degree Reiki for the rest of your life.

Since the Second Degree Reiki attunement literally opens you to all time and all space through the Hon Sha Ze Sho Nen symbol, I suggest taking time after the attunement to contemplate your own eternal nature through meditation, writing poetry, or whatever form works for you personally.

10

Basic Uses of
Second Degree Reiki

Second Degree Reiki has three primary functions: empowering the flow of Reiki with the Cho Ku Rei symbol, directing Reiki to heal mental and emotional issues with the Sei He Ki symbol, and sending Reiki through time and space by using the Hon Sha Ze Sho Nen symbol.

Expansion of Consciousness

Once you have been attuned to Second Degree Reiki, you face an open door. This door is much more than just the raised vibration that happens in your energy field with the attunement; it is also an expanded consciousness. Many Reiki Masters, however, do not teach that Second Degree Reiki expands your consciousness. It does this simply by allowing you to transcend time and space with Reiki. If you use this gift of Second Degree Reiki, how you look at time and space will change.

Unfortunately I know some Second Degree Reiki practitioners who only use it for empowering the flow of Reiki. They seem threatened by the idea of transcending time and space with this energy. I believe this is because they were never taught to allow this expansion in consciousness. In fact, when I was attuned to Second Degree Reiki, this expansion or shift in how I might see the universe was not even mentioned. Reiki is for healing, but sometimes we forget to mention that unbinding our limited view of the universe *is* healing. Often, we only think of healing as undoing the harm caused by physical or emotional trauma. There is much more to healing than just releasing the negatives of life. Healing, in fact, is most potent when it emphasizes how infinite the possibilities in life really are. Expanding your consciousness through Reiki is something I highly encourage. I will offer some tips on this as we explore all aspects of Second Degree Reiki.

Knowing and Using Symbols

The fundamentals of using Second Degree Reiki involve knowing the symbols, which means being able to visualize them and chant them without a book or cheat sheet. Once Reiki practitioners were not allowed to keep copies of the symbols. They had to memorize them. But recently this tradition has shifted for the better. Now several books on Reiki symbols and their uses have been published. This openness was needed. Still, you should learn the symbols so that you fully internalize them. Think of them as an energy alphabet. Just as with reading, once you have learned the alphabet, a whole new world is opened.

Using Cho Ku Rei in Treatment Sessions

Once you have fully memorized and internalized Cho Ku Rei, the power symbol, experiment with how to use it. In a Reiki session, visualize the symbol on each palm of your hand and mentally chant Cho Ku Rei, Cho Ku Rei, Cho Ku Rei continuously.

Try this on yourself. Simply lay each palm on you stomach, and first allow Reiki to flow without using the symbol. This allows you to compare how Reiki flows without and with the symbol being activated. Wait for about a minute so that your body is entirely familiar with the vibration that is flowing out of your hands. Then visualize the symbol on each palm and mentally chant Cho Ku Rei. You will feel the power of Reiki increase as it flows out of your hands. Do this for a minute or two. Afterward, discontinue using the symbol for a minute or two and just allow Reiki to flow as it would without the symbol. You will notice that the vibration lessens again. Using this simple technique, you can see that the Cho Ku Rei symbol acts almost like the volume control on a radio.

Try using the Cho Ku Rei symbol during an entire self-treatment, for the full duration of the session. The vibration increases dramatically. Some might even find that using it for an entire session is overwhelming.

The reason I suggest you experiment with using it on yourself first is so you know what it feels like when you use it on another person.

Personally I like using Cho Ku Rei for about half of the session. I will use it for a few minutes, and then rest. I repeat this pattern over and over through the session. This pattern of high intensity, followed by lower intensity, followed by high intensity again, is much like the rhythms and cycles we experience in our own body rhythms, as well as the rhythms of the moon and of the seasons. I believe it is more natural than constantly using the symbol during a session, though there might be cases when such intensity is needed. The best thing is to experiment, and discover what your own body likes.

Once you are familiar with using the symbol on yourself, begin to ask others whom you treat if they would like to experience this high-intensity Reiki. Give them the right to make this choice. Never use Reiki symbols on another person unless you have been given permission to do so.

Use Cho Ku Rei on others just as you would on yourself, by visualizing the symbol and chanting it in your head. When using the Cho Ku Rei symbol on another person, pay attention to their breathing and their body language. Usually I notice people going deeper into a space of relaxation. But there have been a few times when I noticed people begin to fidget, as if the Reiki was too intense. At times such as these, it is important either to stop using the symbol in the treatment or ask the person if the Reiki feels too strong. You can either discontinue using it for the rest of the treatment or use it only in small bursts to raise the vibration only for brief periods of time. Always communicate with the person you are working on, either directly or by listening to the signs his or her body gives you. The last thing you want to do is overwhelm a person with too much of a good thing. Reiki is wonderful, but some people cannot handle too much of it in one dose.

As you become familiar with using the Cho Ku Rei symbol on yourself and others, you will also become more familiar with the ebb and flow of Reiki, of when to be intense and when to be subtle. These things cannot be taught in a book; you will learn them by listening to your intuition, and to others.

Using Cho Ku Rei in Daily Life

Cho Ku Rei is wonderful to use in sessions, but it can also be a powerful tool in daily life. Drawing the symbol over your food is a quick way to empower your food with positive vibrations. This can be done over beverages as well. In either case, simply draw the symbol in the air over the food or beverage about to be consumed and mentally chant Cho Ku Rei.

A similar technique can be used to clear negative energy from a room or given area. Simply walk around the room in a circle drawing Cho Ku Rei in the air. I make sweeping gestures, drawing the symbol as large as possible. I walk around the room, drawing the symbol over each wall, window, and doorway. I go until I have created an invisible circle of Cho Ku Rei symbols that, if you could see them all, would look like a chain around the entire room. Once the circle is completed, I draw one above my head and one over the floor. All of this time, I am mentally chanting Cho Ku Rei.

Chanting the symbol is something you can do out loud or internally. It can actually be quite fun if you get into a musical rhythm with it. The reason I say to chant it mentally is that I want you to realize that it does not have to be audible. And sometimes chanting the name of the symbol out loud would be socially awkward. Use your own judgment, but know that either way is effective.

Brief Review of Using Cho Ku Rei

In review, using the Cho Ku Rei symbol in a physical treatment on yourself or another simply involves visualizing the symbol and chanting it. That's all. It will increase the flow of Reiki during a treatment. Other uses include drawing the symbol in the air and chanting it to clear away negative vibrations in a room. You can also draw it and chant it over things you eat and drink, to empower them with love and light.

Using Sei He Ki in Mental Healing for Yourself

Sei He Ki is the next symbol you will want to explore. Like Cho Ku Rei, you can use it in a hands-on session with yourself or someone else.

To use Sei He Ki in a mental healing on yourself, simply hold your hands so that your palms are on top of your crown chakra, at the very top of your head. Visualize both Cho Ku Rei and Sei He Ki on the palms of both of your hands, as Cho Ku Rei is what empowers Sei He Ki. Then chant the symbols in repetitions of three such that Cho Ku Rei comes both before and after Sei He Ki, like this:

Cho Ku Rei, Cho Ku Rei, Cho Ku Rei,
Sei He Ki, Sei He Ki, Sei He Ki,
Cho Ku Rei, Cho Ku Rei, Cho Ku Rei

Continue the chant for as long as you wish the mental healing Reiki to flow. You might notice a change in the vibration of the Reiki, as if it were going into the core of your soul. That is exactly what it is doing, going to the soul root of your emotional or mental issue. I have found that doing mental healing Reiki for fifteen minutes a day can clear up some of the most tangled emotional webs I have ever experienced.

Intent is very important in how Sei He Ki is used. If the intent is for general well-being on an emotional level, that is what the Reiki will strive for. You will feel that shift in you emotionally. If the desire is something more specific, like clearing up relationship issues or feelings of stress or anxiety about a particular aspect of your life, this form of Reiki will illuminate those issues so that they become more clear for you to deal with. Just set your intention so that the Reiki knows what to clear up for you mentally. Remember, Reiki has an intelligence that is of a Divine source. It will find the answer to your problem, or at least illuminate the situation so you can make your own clear choices.

Using Sei He Ki in Mental Healing for Others

Once you have used Sei He Ki on yourself a number of times, let people to whom you give Reiki know that they now have the option for receiving mental healing with Reiki. Do not push this on anyone, or try to change people with Reiki. That would be manipulative. Just let them know that this kind of healing is available to them. And if it is in accordance with their own free will, they will ask you for a mental healing when the time is right.

When doing a mental Reiki healing on someone else, ask the person first if there is a specific emotional issue that he or she wants cleared up. If so, intend that the Reiki flow clear this issue, while visualizing the symbols and chanting them appropriately. You do not need to know the exact details, since you are not playing therapist in this role. The person may indicate a desire for Reiki for healing of a relationship issue, family issue, and so on. It is not up to you to sort it out for the person; the Reiki will do that work on its own. If the person has no specific intent, simply use the symbols and let the Reiki flow for the person's general mental well-being.

Using Sei He Ki for Protection

Besides being used for mental healing, Sei He Ki can be used to invoke energies of protection. I tend to use this symbol when clearing a room before Reiki attunements, to add protection from any form of negativity entering the room. Simply use the same method for clearing a room as given above, but add the Sei He Ki symbol in between each Cho Ku Rei as you draw and chant the invisible chain of symbols around the room. You can also draw it over specific objects that you wish to protect, using it in conjunction with Cho Ku Rei so that the protection is activated. Once while apartment searching and without a real home, I used it to protect all my belongings that were in a car parked on the street for over a month in a crime-ridden part of San Francisco. Other cars nearby were being broken into quite often, but my belongings and the car were left unharmed, even though it was clear that the car was full of goodies that could easily have been taken by simply smashing a window. Though I have used the protective aspects less often in direct treatments on individuals, there have been a few times when I drew the symbol over a person's entire body when I sensed the person might be in some kind of danger.

Brief Review of Using Sei He Ki

In review, Sei He Ki can be used for mental healing or for protective purposes. To use it in a mental healing, place your palms over the crown chakra at the top of the head of the person you are working on, while visualizing Sei He Ki in conjunction with Cho Ku Rei. At the same time, chant Cho Ku Rei three times, then Sei He Ki three times, then Cho Ku Rei three times. Repeat this for as long as you wish the mental healing Reiki to flow.

For protection, chant Sei He Ki and draw it in the air over whatever it is you wish to protect. Follow this with drawing and chanting Cho Ku Rei to activate the protection.

Using Hon Sha Ze Sho Nen to Transcend Time and Space

Using Sei He Ki and Cho Ku Rei greatly enhances the abilities you have with Reiki. Now it is possible for you not only to give the healing energy of Reiki to yourself and others, but also to use it for specific purposes such as mental healing or clearing a room of negative vibrations. These two symbols should become part of your very being, such that you feel ready to use them whenever you need. Yet as wonderful as these two symbols are, they cannot be used to their full potential until one masters the use of Hon Sha Ze Sho Nen.

Hon Sha Ze Sho Nen is the symbol that allows you to transcend time and space with Reiki. I strongly encourage you to experiment with the use of this symbol, as it can unlock many secrets about the nature of who we are in relationship to all things. I have used this symbol not only to send healing back in time to traumatic events I experienced in this life, but also to investigate the nature of my own soul. I have used this symbol to send Reiki back to when my soul was first created, to the first instant of my eternal existence. I cannot describe what that feels like or what I learned. It is something I encourage you to investigate on your own.

Since Reiki can be sent to relationships in Second Degree, I have used this symbol to send Reiki to my relationship with the Divine, to heal wounds of my soul, and to come to a greater understanding of the mystery of life. The opportunities to use this symbol to investigate the universe and bring love and light to all aspects of your existence are truly infinite. If you want to know what life was like when you were in the womb, send yourself Reiki backward in time to when you were in the womb. Not only are you healing your own deepest inner child, but you are also coming to know yourself, which is the greatest healing of all. I do not exaggerate when I say that the possibilities for using Second Degree to explore your soul, your past, your past lives, and your relationship to all things is truly infinite. This is the greatest gift Reiki can offer you, and it is one that is often overlooked.

Sending Reiki in Present Time

The fundamentals for using Hon Sha Ze Sho Nen are simple. Think of the symbol as a link through time and space to anywhere at any time of all creation. If you want to send Reiki to a person in present time and have gotten their permission beforehand, simply say that person's name three times, then say Hon Sha Ze Sho Nen three times while visualizing the symbol over the person's face, image, or name. Repeat this several times to establish a strong link. Once the link feels clear, start using Cho Ku Rei to activate Reiki flowing to the person through this link. Continue using Cho Ku Rei, visualizing the symbol and chanting it while sensing the Reiki flow to the intended person. At some point you will probably feel the link begin to fade, as if the presence of the person you are sending Reiki to seems out of reach. When this happens, simply start using Hon Sha Ze Sho Nen again to reconnect the link through time/space. Continue using Cho Ku Rei once the link is strong again.

Sending Reiki in Past or Future Time

If you are sending a Reiki treatment anywhere other than the present, indicate that in the beginning. Simply state out loud the time, which can be future as well as past, when the Reiki is intended to arrive. If you do not know the time, link the arrival of the Reiki to a specific action. For example, send a treatment to your friend forward in time to arrive when they go to bed the next night. You might not know what time they will go to bed, but just state out loud when beginning the treatment that the Reiki is to arrive "at bedtime tomorrow." Otherwise, the treatment technique is exactly the same as shown above.

Some people feel more secure using a photograph, drawing, or doll to represent the person to whom they are sending Reiki. It helps them to visualize the person. They place their hands on the doll or photo, and use the symbols as shown above. Personally I prefer to let myself stay with mental visualization. But if using a doll or photograph helps, then do not hesitate to incorporate that into your technique. One thing that seems pretty universal about Reiki is that it adapts to people, thus allowing for numerous ways to send Reiki that are all correct. Again, I encourage you to experiment and do what feels most comfortable to you.

Brief Review of Using Hon Sha Ze Sho Nen

In review, Hon Sha Ze Sho Nen is used to deliver Reiki to any point on the time/space matrix. To use the symbol, simply say the name of the person or situation you are sending Reiki to three times, and then begin chanting Hon Sha Ze Sho Nen and visualizing the symbol over the designated target for the Reiki treatment. This establishes the link through which the Reiki can flow. To activate the flow of Reiki through this link, begin visualizing and chanting Cho Ku Rei. If the intent of the Reiki arrival is in the past or future, include that when stating the designated target three times in the beginning.

The Power of Second Degree Reiki

Overall, Second Degree Reiki can empower the Reiki flow, clear away negative vibrations, promote mental healing, invoke protective energies, and allow you to transcend time and space with Reiki. While doing that, it can bring you closer to the Divine and provide a means for exploring your relationship to all things. For most people, that is a big shift in consciousness to deal with. Do not feel pressured to get it all at once. The information in this chapter might take some time to mentally digest and integrate. Take your time and review the information in this chapter, or in other Reiki books, as often as necessary. Give yourself the space and time necessary to integrate this new information and how you can best use it in your own life. Your journey into the world of Reiki has just begun.

11

Simple Exercises for
Sending Reiki

Theory is one thing, but only through practice will you come to understand Reiki and how it works. Below are some practice exercises to help you become more proficient in your use of Second Degree Reiki.

Protecting the Earth

For our first exercise, let's send protective Reiki to the earth as an example of how to use all three symbols in a long-distance treatment. If you wish to visualize this Reiki going to a particular area of the earth that you feel needs protection, like the ozone or the redwoods, then do so. Otherwise, you can visualize our blue planet Mother as seen in NASA photographs. Once you have the image of the earth, or the particular region where you wish the healing to go, say the following while visualizing the symbols as you chant:

Earth, Earth, Earth
Hon Sha Ze Sho Nen, Hon Sha Ze Sho Nen, Hon Sha Ze Sho Nen
Cho Ku Rei, Cho Ku Rei, Cho Ku Rei
Sei He Ki, Sei He Ki, Sei He Ki
Cho Ku Rei, Cho Ku Rei, Cho Ku Rei

Repeat the Cho Ku Rei and Sei He Ki parts until the link fades, and then return to chanting "Earth" and Hon Sha Ze Sho Nen to reestablish the link. Do this for five minutes or longer just to get a feel for it.

Bringing World Peace

Another worthy cause for sending Reiki is to help bring world peace. One treatment is obviously not going to do the trick, but one of the great things about Reiki is that it works on all levels. This treatment you are about to send might not prevent the next war, but it will add to the cosmic fabric of peace that desperately wants to engulf this planet. Perhaps one day, if enough of us take this kind of thing seriously, we will have peace on earth. Like the Divine, Reiki can work in mysterious ways.

To do this exercise, simply visualize what you think the world would look like if world peace existed in the present. Then say:

I send this treatment out into the world to help manifest world peace:
World peace, world peace, world peace,
Hon Sha Ze Sho Nen, Hon Sha Ze Sho Nen, Hon Sha Ze Sho Nen
Cho Ku Rei, Cho Ku Rei, Cho Ku Rei
Cho Ku Rei, Cho Ku Rei, Cho Ku Rei

Repeat Cho Ku Rei until you sense a need to use Hon Sha Ze Sho Nen again. Send the treatment for five minutes or more so you get a sense of the experience. You could also include Sei He Ki if you wanted to protect against war. It is simply a matter of how you phrase it and how you want to target the Reiki. If you wish, go back and repeat the above exercise using Sei He Ki as well, adding it between the two lines of Cho Ku Rei.

Returning Blessings to the Divine

As mentioned in chapter 3, Reiki was used in Atlantis. In some cases the people of Atlantis misused it, but in other ways they had a more expanded view of how Reiki could work. For example, they used Reiki to return blessings to the Divine. Does the Divine need this? Probably not, but a thoughtful act like this brings us closer to the Divine. To do this exercise, think of the name that you use for the Divine. Then send Reiki, just as you would send it to a human being. You might notice the infinite presence of the Divine. This experience is truly one that all people should have the right to explore.

12

Alternate Reiki Symbols

Historically, according to the lineage as it came through Hawaya Takata to the West, only three symbols were taught in Second Degree Reiki. Recently many Reiki Masters have been channeling in new symbols. Some people disclaim these as not really being part of the Reiki energy system. I disagree, having used a number of these new symbols and experienced their power and healing ability. They only seem to work in the context of Reiki, and Reiki seems enhanced as an overall system by their inclusion. I consider them to be as much a part of Reiki as Cho Ku Rei or Hon Sha Ze Sho Nen. Reiki is a flexible system that evolves and grows in accordance with our own ability to comprehend it. These new symbols are coming to us now because we are ready for them, and because the earth is desperately in need of accelerated forms of healing. Some of these symbols have been published in books. I highly recommend Diane Stein's book *Essential Reiki* (Berkeley, CA: Crossing Press, 1995) for information about some of these alternate symbols. Other lesser known Reiki Masters are channeling in new symbols as well, teaching them to their students and to other Reiki Masters.

I have chosen to include in this chapter some new symbols that I have channeled in as well. Realize that no one person has all the answers to what Reiki is or knows which symbols are truly part of the Reiki energy system. If the symbols work and rely upon other Reiki symbols to be activated, then they must be Reiki symbols. Again, I encourage you to experiment and arrive at your own conclusions.

Exploring Alternate Symbols

Each symbol that I have listed includes with it a chant for attunement. These symbols are only ones that I have channeled in. I encourage you to explore symbols channeled in by others, as I can personally vouch for their healing ability in many cases. I have not included those other symbols for two reasons: first, I see no need to duplicate what is already written in other books, and, second, I do not claim to be all-inclusive in my investigation of alternate Reiki symbols, and do not want to give the impression that all new Reiki symbols can be found in this book. I am sure there are many symbols that I have not yet experienced that are profoundly useful in the Reiki energy system. My responsibility to teach Reiki in as clean a way as I can means I teach what I know directly. Therefore, only the symbols I have channeled are included here.

Fling Fling

The first alternate symbol I channeled in is called Fling Fling. It looks like and is energetically related to Sei He Ki, but has a slightly different function. This symbol centers and grounds one emotionally and helps disperse unwelcome energetic influences. It should be used in instances where one is experiencing emotional shock, trauma, confusion, or any other form of feeling off balance due to external influences or events. The symbol works on two levels: one is to clear the mental and emotional fields of interference, and the other is simply to ground and center the person on the mental and emotional level. The name implies flinging off something negative, which is what this symbol does. But it also functions in terms of emotional grounding.

This symbol is easy to chant and easy to draw. On the following page is a diagram of how it should be drawn.

To use this symbol on yourself, use it the same way as you would Sei He Ki (see chapter 10). This symbol is more effective than Sei He Ki when it comes to stabilizing and grounding one emotionally, and it works as a filter to disperse those energies that can be the source of one feeling emotionally unbalanced. I use Fling Fling in cases where someone is experiencing emotional confusion, immediate trauma, or shock, whereas Sei He Ki is more effective for healing past emotional wounds and creating an overall feeling of mental and emotional well-being.

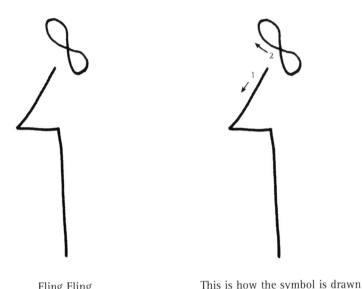

Fling Fling   This is how the symbol is drawn

Before saying the Attunement Chant, agree to do an act of good works in exchange for this gift of the new symbol being activated in your energy field. Once you are attuned to this symbol, I suggest sending three hours of Fling Fling Reiki toward releasing destabilizing energetic influences from the earth. Using this symbol toward war-torn regions of the planet is highly recommended, considering how much emotional shock and trauma exist in such regions of the earth.

Just as with the other attunements, take the necessary steps to make this a sacred occasion. Take your sea-salt bath in the morning. Go to your sacred space. Light candles if you wish, to Dr. Usui and the Divine, and then proceed with asking for the attunement. When you are ready, repeat the following chant:

Blessed be the Ones who brought us Reiki
Blessed be the Ones who continue this sacred light
I ask for the attunement of Fling Fling Reiki
For both First and Second Degree
Blessings unto all
Blessings unto me

Again, use the symbol exactly like Sei He Ki (see chapter 10), but for the purpose of emotional grounding and filtering out destabilizing influences instead of using it for overall mental health. Sei He Ki can help with filtering out destabilizing influences, but Fling Fling seems more Divinely designed for this purpose while also having an emotional grounding function.

Rish Tea

Another symbol I have channeled is called Rish Tea. I have been told that it is strictly for helping focus Reiki more clearly in the battle against cancer. I do not suggest that it is a cure, nor would I recommend anyone abandoning professional medical treatment in favor of this symbol. As with all forms of Reiki, it spiritually complements other healing modalities and is not intended to draw anyone away from other healing sources. Below is a diagram of the symbol.

The attunement, like all others in this book, requires an energy exchange. Since the attunement is activated for both First and Second Degree levels, I suggest sending three hours of Rish Tea Reiki to a major industrial area, to help release the cancer energy as a whole from the places where cancer usually begins.

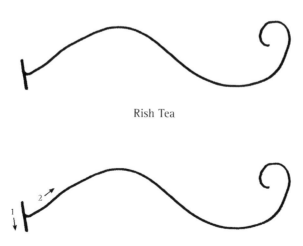

Rish Tea

This is how the symbol is drawn

Another valid means of doing an energy exchange would be to offer Rish Tea Reiki to anyone you might know with cancer, but be careful not to invade anyone's health boundaries. Also be clear that Reiki is a spiritual tool intended to enhance and complement professional medical treatment. It is not intended to be a replacement for professional medical care. Cancer is a very painful issue, as those suffering from the disease are often taunted with possible cures that frequently fail. These experiences torment those in search of true healing. Be aware that some people may feel what you are offering is no different than snake oil. We must make this form of Reiki available to those with cancer without trying to overtake their healing process or pretend that we know what is best for them. Make the offer gently, and then let the person decide for themselves.

Once you have decided on your commitment, make time for your sacred day of being attuned to this symbol. By now, you will have become familiar with the process. Take your sea-salt bath in the morning. Go to your sacred space. Light candles if you wish, to Dr. Usui and the Divine, and then proceed with asking for the attunement by repeating the chant below:

Blessed be the Ones who brought us Reiki
Blessed be the Ones who continue this sacred light
I ask for attunement of Rish Tea Reiki
For both First and Second Degree
Blessings unto all
Blessings unto me

Having now been attuned to this form of Reiki, use the symbol in conjunction with Cho Ku Rei for physical treatments. Once again, Cho Ku Rei is what activates most other symbols. You can use Rish Tea in a full-body session for spiritual preventative purposes on anyone. And if you are working on a person who has cancer, you should combine working the hand positions of a full-body treatment with working on the area where the cancer is located.

Try using this symbol on yourself to get the feel of the energy, which often vibrates slightly hotter or more intensely than most forms of Reiki. Place your palms on your abdomen and allow Reiki to flow without any symbols. Then use the Cho Ku Rei symbol (see chapter 8) and Rish Tea together, visualizing both on your palms while chanting each in sets of three as shown below:

Cho Ku Rei, Cho Ku Rei, Cho Ku Rei
Rish Tea, Rish Tea, Rish Tea
Cho Ku Rei, Cho Ku Rei, Cho Ku Rei

Do this for five minutes to fully feel what the energy is like. Then discontinue using Rish Tea, and use only Cho Ku Rei so you can feel how they are different.

Understanding these symbols as energy, how they feel to the touch, is as important as having an intellectual understanding of them. In a treatment, your hands do the thinking and your mind gets out of the way. This is why I encourage comparing how the symbols feel, so that your hands understand how they are different on a sensory level.

Use Rish Tea for your own health and for helping those around you. But remember, do not push it on anyone. Your offer is all that is necessary.

One Love

The next symbol is one of my favorites. It brings in an energy of deep universal love that feels beyond anything I have experienced energetically. It is called One Love. It has no specific healing focus other than to bring in the energy of love, which can often be the most powerful healer of all. I have used it for myself when feeling low, unloved, or emotionally lost. It always reminds me how deep the power of love is, and how holy all of us are in having the capacity to give and receive this love. It takes me into a space that is whole, no matter what I might be struggling with at the time. I find using it for others can help when they are feeling unloved or emotionally insecure. It is almost like that cosmic teddy bear all of us need to hug once in a while.

For the attunement energy exchange for this symbol, I recommend sending three hours of One Love Reiki to a prison or jail, anyplace where the vibration of love seems almost entirely absent. Remember, you are not sending love to the prisoners, for that would require their consent. You are sending love to the building, the system of interactions, the overall vibration of the prison itself. The point of this is to bring in

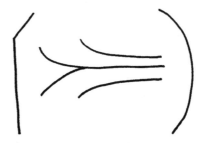

One Love

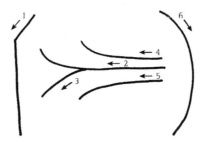

This is how the symbol is drawn

the vibration of love, which will hopefully help the prisoners and the guards interact more humanely, and evolve further toward an atmosphere of compassion and responsibility. You are not trying to heal the individuals, but are trying to shift the vibration such that those who wish to heal will be encouraged to step forward in that direction. Just as with other suggested treatments, I realize that one session might not change much. But when combined with numerous treatments over time, the changes can be stunning.

If this treatment does not feel appropriate for you and your energy exchange, do some other act of good works that feels like a worthy commitment. Once you have decided upon your commitment, prepare for the attunement: choose your day and space, take your sea-salt bath, and light your candles, if that feels right. Then say the following chant to become attuned to One Love Reiki at both the First Degree and Second Degree:

Blessed be the Ones who brought us Reiki
Blessed be the Ones who continue this sacred light
I ask for the attunement of One Love Reiki
For both First and Second Degree
Blessing unto all
Blessings unto me

You might want to really sit with this one after you are attuned, as the vibration of this attunement is very special. But when you are ready, go forward with using this symbol on yourself and others. Just like Sei He Ki, Fling Fling, and Rish Tea, the symbol needs to be empowered with Cho Ku Rei to be activated in a session. In using this symbol you will come to understand how right The Beatles were when they said, "All you need is love."

Rebirth

Rebirth is the name of the next symbol we will examine. Like the name implies, this symbol helps one move through old patterns to be reborn into a new awareness. It is a fantastic symbol to use when life feels stuck, and everything feels faded and old. What I have discovered in using it is that it really helps open doors to new ways of seeing old problems. It is also good to use during transition periods in life.

During the time when I channeled this symbol, my girlfriend at the time also channeled in the same symbol, but as an artistic design she

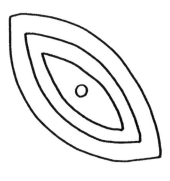

Rebirth

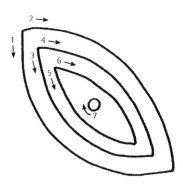

This is how the symbol is drawn

was using in her pottery. I was amazed to notice how both of us were changing during this time in our lives. It was also interesting to see a symbol that had come to me in meditations also appearing on the jars and vases that she was making at the time. She did not know that this symbol had come to me, as I had not shared it with her before she started using it in her artwork. We eventually parted ways, but not before being entirely reborn on the paths in which we had been dabbling in beforehand.

To use this symbol, simply empower it with Cho Ku Rei. I suggest sending three hours of Rebirth Reiki to our national health-care system, to encourage a new awareness that allows all people proper health care, and which does not discount the importance of alternative healing modalities. Again, this is just a suggestion, and you are free to do other acts of good works to complete your energy exchange.

The attunement process is probably quite familiar to you by now. Below is the attunement chant for Rebirth Reiki. Once you say this chant, you will be attuned to First and Second Degree Reiki of this symbol.

Blessed be the Ones who brought us Reiki
Blessed be the Ones who continue this sacred light
I ask for the attunement of Rebirth Reiki
For First and Second Degree
Blessings unto all
Blessings unto me

Once you are attuned, use this symbol for helping yourself or others move smoothly through life transitions, or times when you are feeling stuck.

One Light

This symbol is helpful for all situations, as it illuminates and opens the door to universal light. It is called One Light.

Use this symbol with the same technique used for all alternate symbols, by empowering it with Cho Ku Rei. The energy exchange for the attunement to this symbol should be three hours of Reiki toward any worthy or selfless cause. Remember, just sending Reiki for your own

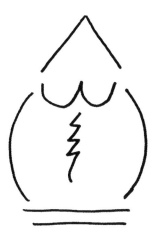

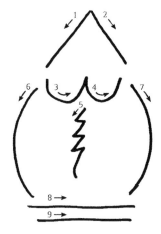

One Light   This is how the symbol is drawn

situation or healing does not constitute an energy exchange. The idea is to give selflessly. Let your own inner guide tell you where to send Reiki as an energy exchange for being attuned to this symbol.

Being familiar with the attunement process, you will know by now what suits you as far as making the day and space sacred to you. When the time is right, say the following chant to be attuned to One Light Reiki:

> *Blessed be the Ones who brought us Reiki*
> *Blessed be the Ones who continue this sacred light*
> *I ask for the attunement of One Light Reiki*
> *For both First and Second Degree*
> *Blessings unto all*
> *Blessings unto me*

Relax and allow the beauty of this experience to encompass you. Use this symbol as you will to bring more light into your world and into the lives of those who are willing to have you use this symbol when performing treatments for them.

Open the Mountain from the Inside

Open the Mountain from the Inside is used for releasing obstacles to learning and freedom. I have found it quite useful in my own graduate studies, and in allowing myself to be more open to what comes to me in the metaphysical realm. Use it as you would the other symbols, by empowering it with Cho Ku Rei.

I suggest sending a three-hour session of Reiki with this symbol to our education system, which has many obstacles to learning and freedom. As with the other symbols, do what is necessary as far as finding a sacred time and space for the attunement, cleansing your aura, and lighting candles if you wish. Below is the attunement chant for this symbol:

Blessed be the Ones who brought us Reiki
Blessed be the Ones who continue this sacred light
I ask for the attunement of
Open the Mountain from the Inside Reiki
For First and Second Degree
Blessings unto all
Blessings unto me

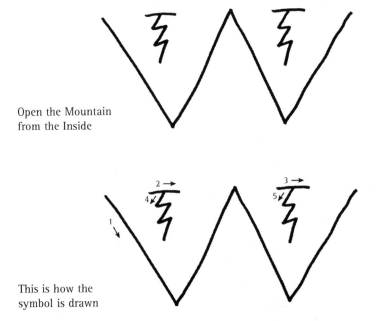

Open the Mountain
from the Inside

This is how the
symbol is drawn

Use this symbol for yourself to help release your own limitations. Use it in your community for helping schools and all centers of learning to be emotionally open and intellectually free institutions.

Mary and the Three Virgins

I channeled in this symbol from Mother Mary. Mary and the Three Virgins is used to bring a sense of being consoled, of knowing that you are not alone in your struggles. Like the other symbols, it is empowered by using Cho Ku Rei before and after. The vibration of it is very smooth, very loving.

The suggested energy exchange for this symbol is to send three hours of Reiki using this symbol to a part of the world that seems troubled. This will shift from time to time, but the Middle East is usually a good place to start. Inner cities, ghettos, homeless shelters are also places that can benefit from this energy. Use your own inner guidance to determine the best place to send this treatment, or do some other good work that feels

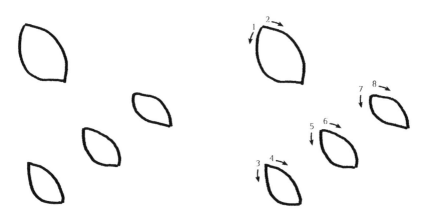

Mary and the Three Virgins   This is how the symbol is drawn

correct. Treat this occasion of the attunement as sacred, and do what is necessary to make the most of that day. Below is the attunement chant:

Blessed be the Ones who brought us Reiki
Blessed be the Ones who continue this sacred light
I ask for the attunement of
Mary and the Three Virgins Reiki
For both First and Second Degree
Blessings unto all
Blessings unto me

Use this symbol whenever you or anyone else you know is in a time of trouble or despair.

Mezzerenthra

Mezzerenthra is used for enhancing your connection to Reiki and the source of Reiki. It is a symbol that can be used to further and deepen your Reiki path.

For the energy exchange for this symbol, I suggest sending a three-hour treatment to humanity as a whole, that it may deepen its connection to Reiki. But again, other acts of good works can serve as your energy exchange. Do what you need to create your sacred time and

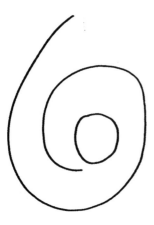

Mezzerenthra

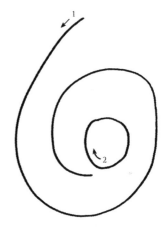

This is how the symbol is drawn

space for receiving the attunement, and when you are ready say this attunement chant:

> *Blessed be the Ones who brought us Reiki*
> *Blessed be the Ones who continue this sacred light*
> *I ask for the attunement of Mezzerenthra Reiki*
> *For both First and Second Degree*
> *Blessings unto all*
> *Blessings unto me*

Use this symbol for deepening your spiritual connection to Reiki, and for making Reiki a greater part of your life.

Symbols for Clearing Chakras

The next seven symbols—one for each chakra—are used for clearing the chakras. To use them, simply empower the symbols with Cho Ku Rei while working on or near the chakra you are intending to clear. Using this system of symbols can be a great way to balance your energy field and maintain good health both emotionally and physically. I recommend doing a short treatment on each chakra every day, just for a few minutes. The symbols are below, and the chant follows after the seventh symbol.

Om Shee Nu Va (root chakra)

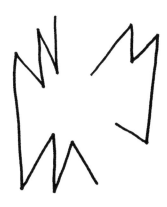

Om Shee Nu Va

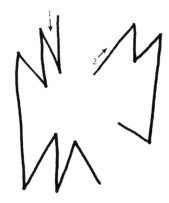

This is how the symbol is drawn

Kali Yoni (sex and emotions chakra)

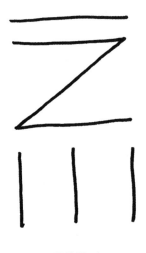

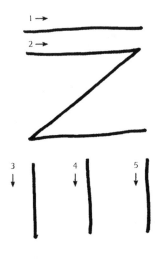

Kali Yoni   This is how the symbol is drawn

Va Shna Hei (power chakra)

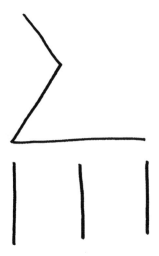

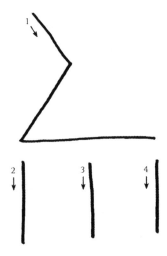

Va Shna Hei   This is how the symbol is drawn

Sama Dee Nah (heart chakra)

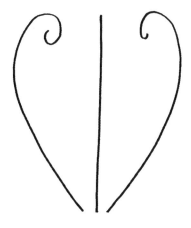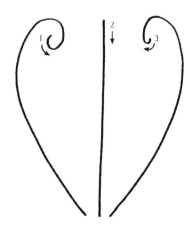

Sama Dee Nah   This is how the symbol is drawn

Ushta Rollo Veh (throat chakra)

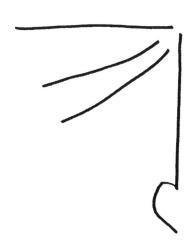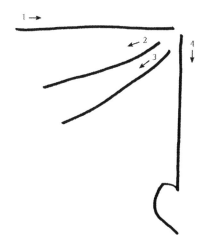

Ushta Rollo Veh   This is how the symbol is drawn

Brahma Vo (third-eye chakra)

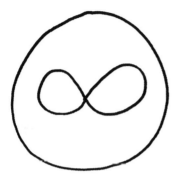

Brahma Vo

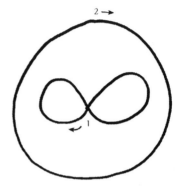

This is how the symbol is drawn

So Mah Kee (crown chakra)

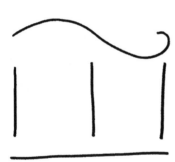

So Mah Kee

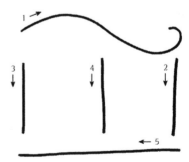

This is how the symbol is drawn

For the energy exchange, use your own discernment. Do some good work that feels right. Though there are seven symbols in this group, I do not think that you should do twenty-one hours of Reiki because of that. The symbols work as a group, so sending five hours of Reiki toward a worthy cause would be right. Use your own judgment on this.

Do what is necessary to set the sacred space for yourself, and then say the attunement chant below:

Blessed be the Ones who brought us Reiki
Blessed be the Ones who continue this sacred light
I ask for the attunement of Reiki of the following symbols:
Om Shee Nu Va, Kali Yoni, Va Shna Hei, Sama Dee Nah
Ushta Rollo Veh, Brahma Vo, So Mah Kee
To both First and Second Degree
Blessings unto all
Blessings unto me

Use these seven symbols to maintain balance and harmony in your daily life.

13

Third Degree Reiki Symbols

In Third Degree Reiki, you are attuned and trained with the capacity to attune others to Reiki. Again, I do not intend this book as a guide for professional training. It takes quite a lot of patience and intuitive skill to be a good Reiki Master. If you wish for that kind of path, then get proper training so that you fully understand issues that are not explored in this book. Being a Reiki Master requires an understanding of human psychology and soul development that cannot be learned from reading a book. I strongly urge you just to use this information for yourself, and for your own healing. Becoming attuned at this level will allow you the freedom to fully explore Reiki as a means for changing your own life. This is what is intended in giving you this information. There might be some who will misuse what is being offered here. I offer such individuals this warning: do not misuse or misrepresent this Divine energy, for the consequences are severe negative karma.

I put forth this information with the hope and belief that it will ultimately help humanity undergo the changes necessary for manifesting a world that is a true Utopia. My efforts in this are sincere, though I realize this will also radically change the world of Reiki.

Things that I wish to explore with offering Third Degree Reiki in this book involve techniques that will allow one to release attunements as well as give them. That is something most Reiki Masters are not aware of. I have also developed techniques for attuning food, candles, body parts, and running cords of Reiki through the time/space matrix that have the power to greatly accelerate the human capacity for healing. There are also ways to attune stones to Reiki and to use them for healing. If science finds a way to tap this vibration of energy that comes out of the stones, humanity will have an energy supply that would be infinite, as the stones flow Reiki constantly. In offering Third Degree to all humanity, I hope the impact will be a revolution in human science and consciousness. I cannot see withholding this information any longer, and only trust that the Divine will be our guide in how this information is used. With this understanding, let us go forward with examining the symbols of Third Degree Reiki.

Tibetan Master Symbol (Daikomyo)

The first symbol we will look at is referred to as the Tibetan Master symbol. Since some people trace Reiki back to Tibet, that is where it gets its name. The symbol is also called Daikomyo, as is another symbol. Daikomyo means "Great Being of the Universe, shine on me, be my friend." The uses of both Daikomyo symbols embody the energy and meaning of that phrase. The Tibetan Master symbol is used to pass the Reiki attunement through the crown chakra in a technique called "the violet breath."

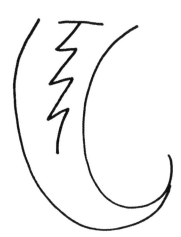

Tibetan Master symbol

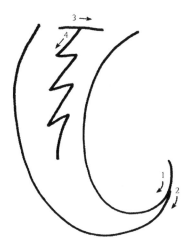

This is how the symbol is drawn

Usui Master Symbol (Daikomyo)

The second symbol that is also referred to as Daikomyo is the Usui Master symbol. It is used in the attunement process as well, and can empower other symbols in the same fashion as Cho Ku Rei but with a higher intensity.

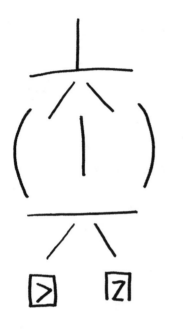

Usui Master symbol

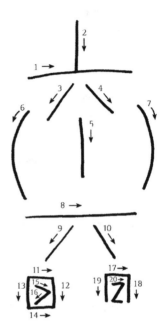

This is how the symbol is drawn

Raku (Fire Dragon)

The third symbol that is learned in Third Degree Reiki is called Raku. Some other Reiki Masters refer to it as Fire Dragon. It is used for opening the aura during the attunement process.

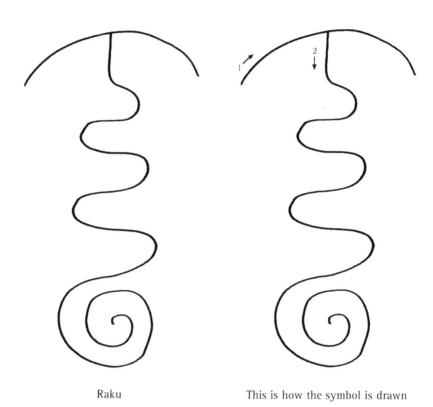

Raku   This is how the symbol is drawn

Using Third Degree Reiki Symbols

How to use the Third Degree Reiki symbols is something that you must learn in the context of learning the Reiki attunement process. This shall be explored further on in chapter 17. For now, it is important to fully memorize the chant and technique for drawing each symbol. Practice daily until you can draw and chant each symbol effortlessly.

14

Third Degree Reiki Attunement

One of the most sacred experiences I ever have had in this life was being attuned to Third Degree Reiki. For days afterward, I felt an extreme connection to the Divine and an awareness of the holiness that exists in all things. It was beautiful.

I have heard that simply being attuned to Reiki at the Third Degree helps you become clear on your soul's path and mission in life. Life lessons always come quicker when you become attuned to any level of Reiki, but at the Third Degree, there is a profound shift that occurs at the soul level. Suddenly you notice that things in your life that never made sense before become clear. An understanding will arise, and with that understanding will come the ability to learn your lessons and move further on your evolutionary path.

Energy Exchange for Attunement

The commitment for the energy exchange at this level should be significantly greater than all the others. Though I disagree with the concept of charging $10,000 for this attunement, many people have paid this amount for becoming attuned to Third Degree Reiki. The reality is that the shifts and blessings that come to you with this attunement are priceless. So take this into consideration when performing your act of good works. If you choose to send Reiki as an act of good works, I recommend twelve hours toward a worthy cause such as healing the earth, eliminating racism, or ending world hunger. Obviously you do not need to send all twelve hours at once. Break it up over a period of weeks, sending half-hour or full-hour treatments until you have logged in twelve hours or more.

Preparation for Attunement

As with the other attunements that are offered in this book, you will want to find a sacred space for yourself, take a sea-salt bath, and light candles to Dr. Usui and the Divine, if that feels appropriate. Really make sure that you will have the whole day to yourself, as your consciousness will be opened into new realms with this attunement.

The Attunement Experience

When the day and time are right, say the attunement chant below and become attuned to Third Degree Reiki:

Blessed be the Ones who brought us Reiki
Blessed be the Ones who continue this sacred light
I ask for the attunement of Reiki Third Degree
Blessings unto all
Blessings unto me

Once attuned, take time to really absorb the beauty of what has happened to you. Enjoy this day. Walk in the woods or on the beach. Write poetry. Enjoy the simple beauties of life, which this attunement illuminates by changing your consciousness.

15

Attuning Stones and
Candles to Reiki

Third Degree Reiki is primarily about using the attunement process. To learn how to pass a Reiki attunement, you first need to have the symbols memorized, as I previously mentioned. Also, most people must learn a technique for raising energy during the attunement process. This involves closing energetic gates by contracting the muscle at the Hui Yin, an energy gate between the anus and genitals, and also raising the tongue up to the upper palate behind the teeth, which closes another energy gate, allowing one's energy level to rise up to a higher vibration. Some who are involved in shamanism, magic, or other forms of spiritual energy work before coming to Reiki often have a high enough vibration to pass an attunement without adding anything extra. But most Reiki Masters need time to develop this specific technique.

Raising Your Energy Level

The Hui Yin is a point in acupressure between the anus and genitals. There is a small muscle there called the perineum that can be contracted. When contracting this muscle and also lifting the top of your tongue to the roof of your mouth just behind the teeth, your overall vibration surges to a higher level. It is from this high energy level that the capacity to perform Reiki can be passed from one individual to another during an attunement.

Take some time to practice contracting the muscle at the Hui Yin, while lifting the tongue tip to touch the roof of your mouth, about an inch behind your front teeth. It might take a number of weeks to get good at doing this. You want to achieve a level where you can hold this position for quite a long time; this position is held during the entire attunement process, which can be quite lengthy if done for a group. Once you are proficient at holding this position for a number of minutes, experiment with performing a Reiki attunement on a stone.

Attuning Stones

Stones will emit Reiki once attuned, and I have often used them on myself as Reiki healers from the mineral kingdom. Practicing on stones is something that helps you learn how to pass an attunement to a human—and it creates wonderful healing tools that can be used for yourself or to give to others as gifts.

To begin the attunement process for a stone draw all six of the traditional Second and Third Degree Reiki symbols in the air over the stone. In a human attunement, this is done primarily to protect a person being attuned while their aura is opened up during the attunement, but I suggest using this protective shield when passing attunements on stones as well. It is good to get into the habit of drawing the six symbols for this purpose, beginning with the Tibetan Master symbol, then Raku, then the Usui Master symbol, then Cho Ku Rei, then Sei He Ki, and finally Hon Sha Ze Sho Nen.

Once you have drawn all six traditional symbols in the air, give the universe a mental intent as to whether or not the attunement is for First or Second Degree. (If it is for Third Degree, the attunement process is slightly different.) Now, contract the perineum and raise the tongue to the upper palate behind the teeth (hold this if you can during the entire attunement). Then draw Raku in the air over the stone, which opens it to receive the rest of the Reiki symbols.

At this point, you wait for what is called the violet breath. You will see a violet image of the Tibetan Master symbol in your mind. Once you see this, visualize the symbol appearing in your mouth and then blow it into the stone.

Once the violet breath has occurred and been passed into the stone, draw the Usui Master symbol in the air over the stone and guide it into the stone with your hand, visualizing it penetrating into the center of the stone. Repeat the exact same process now using Cho Ku Rei, drawing the symbol in the air and guiding it into the stone. Then repeat the same process using Sei He Ki. Finish this part of the attunement by drawing Hon Sha Ze Sho Nen over the stone, and guiding it into the stone like the other symbols. If you are adding an alternative symbol, draw it in the air and guide it in at this point like the other symbols. The Raku symbol is the only Reiki symbol not actually guided into the stone; it is only used for opening the stone to receive the symbols.

Next, turn the stone over and draw Cho Ku Rei in the air over the stone. Now, using the same hand you used to draw Cho Ku Rei, tap the stone three times, and mentally chant Cho Ku Rei with each tap. Repeat the same process using Sei He Ki, drawing it in the air once while tapping it into the stone and chanting three times. Repeat the same process using Hon Sha Ze Sho Nen. If adding an alternative symbol, repeat the same process now using the alternative symbol.

Now, hold both hands over the stone, and blow from one end of the stone to the other, then back again.

At this point, I ask mentally for this stone to channel Reiki with Divine love and wisdom. I then seal the process by visualizing three Cho Ku Rei symbols over the stone and mentally say: "This process is sealed with Divine love and light." Then I turn the stone back over, and while releasing the perineum and tongue, I blow one final breath, which is a blessing to the stone that is now attuned to Reiki.

Practice this on as many stones as you like. In a shamanic view of the world, these stones have a consciousness and should be asked if they want to be attuned. In other words, do not just go out and grab any random stone you find and attune it. Send out your intent that you will find the right stone, one that wishes to be attuned. Listening to your intuition, you will be called to a stone that is in agreement with this wish.

Once you have attuned the stone, hold it in your hands and feel the Reiki flowing out of it. (If it is attuned to an alternate symbol, you will feel the energy of that particular symbol.) This is a good way to get confidence that the attunement method works. What else could be causing the stone to emit Reiki except for the attunement? Sometimes when attuning a person to Reiki you might think that maybe it is only a mind trick, that their hands are getting hot because they believe in the attunement. But when working with stones it confirms that the Reiki attunement is valid and real. Keep working with this process of attuning stones until you have full confidence in your ability to pass an attunement. Practice until it is easy and effortless. Use the stones for your own healing by laying them on parts of your body that need Reiki. I often fall into a relaxing sleep when doing this for myself. You can also use the stones in healing others, treating them like an extra hand that is flowing Reiki.

Attuning Candles

Having gained confidence by working with attuning stones to Reiki, it is time to work with attuning candles. The reason I suggest attuning candles is that I have learned that by synthesizing Reiki with candle magic, it is possible to send Reiki for hours or even days at a time to specific situations or for intensive healings. Candle magic empowers candles with spiritual energies, often using oils, herbs, or ritualized markings such as runes, angelic sigils, or planetary signs that are added to the candle to bring about the intended energetic function. In Reiki candle magic, we are simply attuning the candle to Reiki as the primary means of empowering it. I once attuned a candle for a friend who had Lyme disease in the early stages. Penicillin was not getting rid of the disease, nor were alternative methods helping him, not even traditional Reiki treatments. He overcame the illness only after we used a treatment of Reiki-attuned candles to send him intensive healing for seven days straight. This reveals to me how powerful Reiki-attuned candles can be as a healing tool.

When I attune a candle to Reiki, I usually use a large candle that is capable of burning safely for several days. I make sure that when I burn one, I have it in a jar or other glass container that sits in a pool of water. I often use my bathtub for this, filling up the bottom with an inch or two of water and placing the glass container with the candle in the bathtub. If you cannot surround it with water, do not let it burn continuously.

To attune the candle, contract the perineum and raise your tongue to the upper palate while drawing all six traditional Reiki symbols in the air, adding any alternate symbols you are using in this attunement as well. Once this is done, send out your mental intent of what level the attunement is for. (I always use Second Degree in this case, since I intend the candles to send Reiki through the time/space matrix.) Then draw Raku in the air from the top to the bottom of the candle. Now that the candle can receive the symbols, await the violet breath and blow it into the top of the candle, visualizing it going down through the center of the candle. Then draw the Usui Master symbol over the top of the candle, guiding it into the candle with your hand and visualizing it moving into the candle's center. Repeat this with Cho Ku Rei, drawing it over the top, then guiding it with your hand first, and then your mind, into the center of the candle. Repeat this with Sei He Ki. Finally, repeat using the Hon Sha Ze Sho Nen symbol. Add alternate symbols at this point if you wish, using the same process as above.

Once you have placed the symbols in through the top of the candle, turn the candle over and draw Cho Ku Rei in the air over the bottom of the candle. Use the same hand to then tap the bottom three times while chanting Cho Ku Rei with each tap. Repeat the same process with Sei He Ki. Then repeat the exact same process with Hon Sha Ze Sho Nen. Add alternate symbols here if you wish, using the same process as above. After Hon Sha Ze Sho Nen or the last alternate symbol is drawn, tapped, and chanted into the bottom of the candle, blow over the candle from the top to the bottom and back up to the top. Then mentally project the affirmation into the candle that it send Reiki according to Divine love and wisdom. Seal the process with three visualized Cho Ku Rei symbols over the candle and mentally say: "I now seal this process with Divine love and light." Then release the perineum and tongue from their held positions while blowing a blessing over the candle. With the candle attuned, you now have a tool that can send Reiki for hours or even days. In the next chapter, you will be shown how to use this new tool.

16

Using Reiki Stones
and Reiki Candles

In the previous chapter, you were shown how to attune stones and
candles to Reiki. Part of this is so you can practice and become proficient with the attunement process. However, stones and candles that are
attuned to Reiki can be wonderful tools. First, let us look at how to use
stones that are attuned to Reiki.

How to Use Reiki Stones
The great thing about using stones that are attuned to Reiki is that you
can place them on your body and let yourself relax in ways that you
might not be able to when giving yourself a Reiki treatment. The stones
emit Reiki constantly. They don't get tired. They don't charge you by
the hour. If you want Reiki for two or three hours during a time of illness, these stone healers are perfect for such times.

I usually have a large supply of Reiki stones. Some are attuned to
normal Reiki, and others are attuned to alternative symbols. The ones
that are attuned to alternative symbols emit the energy of those symbols
constantly. I usually use only one alternate symbol per stone because of
this, but you can use more if you want those energies combined and
flowing simultaneously.

My favorite way of using a Reiki stone is to place a stone that is
attuned to One Love Reiki over the back of my heart chakra so that I am
able to relax facing down. The stone rests on my back, lying on my mid-
upper spine, flowing One Love Reiki into the back of my heart chakra.
This is a wonderful experience for anyone to have at any time, but it can

also be a healing experience for one who feels unloved or unworthy of love. Just keep the stone there for as long as you like. When you are finished, honor the stone by cleansing it with water and returning it to a special place in your home. I place my Reiki stones near houseplants in my apartment, sometimes even surrounding a plant with Reiki stones in the soil. The plants seem to like it, and so do the stones.

Another nice treatment involves using two stones attuned to traditional Reiki symbols. Place one stone on your tailbone and the other on your neck while lying face down. The Reiki will flow between the stones through your spine. Essentially this is the spine-balancing technique described in the Reiki treatment for others (see chapter 6). However, thanks to the stones you can have this treatment for yourself whenever you wish.

Obviously using stones for self-healing in this way allows you the freedom to totally relax. There is no need to hold your arms in a particular position or to keep alert for what to do next. Simply place the stones where you wish to have Reiki, and relax. If you have a specific condition that needs attention, place several stones in the area that needs healing. For example, a person being treated for cancer may wish to place several stones attuned to Rish Tea Reiki over an area where the cancer is present in the body. A person with a chest cold may wish to place several stones on his or her chest. Again, you are only limited by your imagination and the number of stones available. When you are finished with a treatment from Reiki stones, take off the stones and allow yourself some time to ground. You can do this by doing a few minutes of Reiki on your feet.

A nice way to balance your energy is to simply hold a Reiki stone in each hand for five minutes. As the stones flow Reiki through your arms to each other, you are also flowing Reiki to the stones, which means that Reiki is coming in through your crown and treating the upper half of your body. This happens every time you give Reiki, but having the stones flow Reiki through your arms to each other during this time really amplifies the effect. Holding stones in this manner will leave you feeling calm, clear, and centered.

A final note about using stones for Reiki: I have noticed that the heavier the mass of the stone, the stronger the Reiki seems to flow through it. I prefer having a variety of sizes for different purposes. I have a couple of stones that are flat and cover most of my belly, emitting quite a strong flow of Reiki. I also keep a few small stones that I can place on my forehead and face, but I do not expect to get the same results from the smaller stones. When working with smaller stones, I use several of them in a treatment so that the Reiki among them is amplified. Again, I encourage you to experiment for yourself and come to your own conclusions about what works best for you.

How to Use Reiki Candles

Reiki candles are not as simple to use as Reiki stones, but they have a much greater capacity for promoting significant long-term change with the Reiki that is sent. This is because the Reiki can be sent literally for days at a time. Think of this, if a one-hour treatment can promote well-being, what might a thirty-hour treatment do? The possibility of over-doing it does exist, but when used wisely, a Reiki candle is a very potent means of addressing both physical illness and situational issues.

To use a Reiki candle once you have attuned it, simply write on the candle where the Reiki is intended to be sent. For example, you might write: "This candle sends Reiki to make my week clear, open, and loving." I usually use a felt-tipped pen to write on the glass surrounding the candle, but you can use a small knife or pin to write into the wax if you prefer. Once you have written out the intent, then charge the candle with your own psychic energy by placing one hand over the top of the candle and the other over the bottom of the candle, visualizing the candle filling up with your own psychic fuel. It is this fuel that gives the candle energy to do the work of magic. The magic you are asking it to do is to send Reiki in accordance with your intent. Again, make sure that your intent is for you or for someone who has given permission for your help. Once you have written out your intent and charged the candle, put it in a safe place to burn for hours or days. This means putting it in some container filled with water, with the pool of water wider than the height of the candle. This is so that if the candle falls over, it will be put out by the water. This is absolutely necessary. Any other means, unless you can constantly be in the same room with the candle, are unsafe.

I have used Reiki candles in my own personal healing journey to help release emotional wounds from the past. This is not something I would recommend doing until you are clearly ready for it. It can be emotional and may leave you feeling ungrounded for a number of days. But if you are looking to get to the core of an issue that will not go away, I recommend using a large Reiki candle that can burn for a week without stopping. Often you will find these candles in metaphysical bookstores. Charge the candle to send Sei He Ki for mental healing. Let it burn for a week. Make sure you drink plenty of fluids during this time, as this much Reiki causes your kidneys to work overtime. If you do not drink plenty of water and juice, you will get dehydrated during this kind of treatment, the kind of dehydration which causes headaches. After the week is up, you should notice some deep changes in your own perceptions and emotions about the issue at hand.

Using Reiki candles is excellent for addressing all issues—physical, mental, or situational. Again, you are only limited by your imagination and the free will of others. Reiki candles can be great healers. Use them wisely.

17

Attuning Others to Reiki

The information in this chapter is intended for attuning family members, relatives, friends, and lovers who want to explore further their own experiences with Reiki. (As I have said before, those who wish to become Reiki practitioners need to train fully—in person—with a certified Reiki Master.) I include Reiki attunement information in this book in order to make Reiki an integral part of the human experience and raise the overall vibration of human consciousness.

The Availability of Reiki to All

Attuning a loved one is one of the great joys of life. To be involved in this sacred act with one who is close to you is spiritually enriching beyond measure. I would like all people to be able to have that experience. Also, my spiritual guidance informs me that Reiki is no longer a privilege, but is in fact a right of all humans, an essential part of our continued evolution as a spiritual species. This does not mean we are all to become professional Reiki healers, for that takes time, dedication, and training. But it does mean that Reiki—as a common spiritual energetic language; as a source of healing for self, friends, and family; as a means for deepening our connection to the Divine and those beings with whom we share this planet—is now available to those who wish for it on that level.

Perhaps one day a child receiving a Reiki attunement from a parent will be commonplace, part of growing up and learning about life. Since Reiki symbols are much like an energy alphabet, perhaps becoming literate in this field is something that will happen in all homes. Just as there is power in being literate, there is power in having the ability to shift the energy of a room, a workplace, or a relationship just by knowing symbols and being attuned. This power is currently reserved for the few, mostly the affluent. How great it will be when all people will have these abilities. This is one step in taking humanity into that place.

Imagine how life would have been different if you could have sent Sei He Ki Reiki to prevent negative encounters with bullies as a child. Why shouldn't all people have this ability? Imagine what it would be like to help relieve the pain a friend or loved one experiences from illness or injury. Shouldn't having that capacity be part of our common humanity? Such abilities exist, and we have the capacity now to offer them on a grand scale. The idea that Reiki is reserved for a few only causes separation and leads away from Oneness. The door must be opened to all, even though some might choose to dishonor the intent of this book by claiming to be fully trained Reiki healers when they are not. Those who feel this way are few, and shall become even fewer as all humanity begins to merge with this Divine energy called Reiki.

The First and Second Degree Attunement Process

To begin the attunement process, draw all six Reiki symbols (the Tibetan Master symbol, the Usui Master symbol, Raku, Cho Ku Rei, Sei He Ki, and Hon Sha Ze Sho Nen) in the air while standing behind the person whom you are going to attune. The person should be seated, though that is for convenience and not absolutely required. While drawing the six Reiki symbols in the air for protection, contract the Hui Yin while lifting the tongue to the roof of the mouth. Mentally send out your intention for the attunement to be either First or Second Degree Reiki. Third Degree Reiki attunements are slightly different, and will be shown later.

After you have drawn the symbols in the air, contracted the perineum muscle at the Hui Yin, lifted the tongue to the upper palate, and set the intention, draw Raku in the air from the top of the person's head down to the tailbone, so that the end spiral swirls at the coccyx. This opens the aura of the person to receive the symbols.

Now lean over the back of the person's head so that your mouth is above the top of the head. Mentally ask for the violet breath and wait for it to arrive. When you see it, blow the violet Tibetan Master symbol into the crown chakra of the person, into the top of the head, and visualize it going down to the base of the brain stem, where the skull is joined to the neck.

Next, draw the Usui Master symbol over the person's head and guide it down with your hand, visualizing it going into his or her head and down to the brain stem.

Now tap on the person's shoulder and ask the person to raise his or her hands above the head, with hands together as if in prayer position.

Draw Cho Ku Rei in the air over the hands and top of the head, guiding and visualizing the symbol going through the person's hands and down through the top of the head into the brain stem. Repeat this using Sei He Ki. Repeat this process one last time using Hon Sha Ze Sho Nen. Alternate symbols can be added after Hon Sha Ze Sho Nen, using the same process.

Now come to the front of the person. Gently pull the person's hands out in front so that the palms are open, fingers extended, in front of the torso. Hold one of your hands underneath the person's hands for support, and use the other hand to draw Cho Ku Rei in the air over the person's palms. Mentally chant Cho Ku Rei three times while also tapping his or her palms three times.

Once you have placed Cho Ku Rei into the person's palms, draw Sei He Ki in the air over the palms and mentally chant Sei He Ki three times while tapping the palms with each chant.

Having placed Sei He Ki into the person's palms, repeat the above process using Hon Sha Ze Sho Nen. Afterward, add any alternate symbols using the same process.

Now close the hands together over the chest so that it seems as if the person is praying. At this point, blow over the chakras by going from the top of the head down to the genitals and back up to the top of the head, using one breath if possible.

Once again, move behind the person, placing your hands on the shoulders and repeating the following phrase three times mentally: *May Divine love and wisdom empower you in your use of Reiki.*

Then place your palms at the base of the person's skull, visualizing three Cho Ku Rei symbols going in and sealing the process. While doing this, mentally say: *I now seal this process with Divine love and light.*

Come back in front of the person, and gently guide the person's hands so that one palm is over his or her heart and the other over the abdomen. This allows the person to feel the new gift of Reiki flowing through his or her hands. At this point, release the perineum and tongue while blowing a breath of blessing to the person.

You and the person should be still for a while, letting this sacred moment be with you. Let the person who has just been attuned determine when it is right to let this sacred moment go. Some people sit with it for ten seconds. Others hold that space for what seems like an hour, though it is probably only five or ten minutes.

The Third Degree Attunement Process

To perform a Third Degree Reiki attunement, change just a few things in the attunement process. You start from behind the person, asking the person to raise his or her hands above the head, hands together as if ready to say a prayer. Draw the six traditional Reiki symbols (the Tibetan Master symbol, the Usui Master symbol, Raku, Cho Ku Rei, Sei He Ki, and Hon Sha Ze Sho Nen) in the air and contract the Hui Yin while lifting your tongue tip to touch the roof of your mouth. You can mentally intend that the attunement be for Third Degree, though this is inherent in the fact that you are delivering this style of attunement. Once the symbols are drawn, open the person's aura with Raku drawn from the top of the head down to the tailbone. Now await the violet breath. And when it comes, blow the Tibetan Master symbol down through the person's hands, into his or her head, where it is visualized going to the base of the brain stem. Now draw the Usui Master symbol in the air over the person's hands, and guide it through the person's hands into his or her head, where you visualize it going down to the base of the brain stem. Now draw Raku over the person's hands, guiding it down into his or her head and lodging at the base of the brain stem. Repeat this with Cho Ku Rei and then with Sei He Ki. Finish this part of the attunement by repeating the same process with Hon Sha Ze Sho Nen.

At this point, come to the front of the person and gently pull the person's hands open in front of you so that his or her palms are together facing upward, fingers extended. Draw the Tibetan Master symbol in the air over the palms and tap the palms three times while you chant "Daikomyo" with each tap. Then draw the Usui Master symbol in the air over the person's palms and tap the palms three times while again chanting Daikomyo with each tap. Now draw Raku over the person's palms and tap the palms three times while chanting Raku with each tap.

Repeat the same process with Cho Ku Rei, drawing the symbol, tapping it into the palms, and chanting it. Repeat the same process with Sei He Ki. Finish this part of the attunement by repeating the same process with Hon Sha Ze Sho Nen and blowing on the person from the head, down to their groin, and back up to their head again.

Now go behind the person, placing your hands on his or her shoulders. Three times say mentally: *May Divine love and wisdom guide you in your use of Reiki.*

Now place your palms at the base of the person's skull, visualizing three Cho Ku Rei symbols sealing the process at the brain stem while mentally chanting Cho Ku Rei three times. Then say mentally: *I now seal this process with Divine love and light.*

Once again, come to the front of the person, placing the person's hands so that one palm rests over the heart and the other over the abdomen. Then release the Hui Yin and occipital lift while blowing a blessing onto the person, knowing that he or she is now fully initiated into Third Degree Reiki.

As with any attunement, make sure that there is sacred time and space for the person to fully absorb this moment in all its beauty and wonder.

Requesting an Energy Exchange

With all the Reiki attunements you give, it is important to ask for some kind of energy exchange. This is tricky since I also advocate that you not use this information to attempt being a professional Reiki Master. An energy exchange is needed because people who do not give something back often never really appreciate the gift that they now have. I have attuned some people for free in my life, and each time the person never seemed to fully grasp what Reiki meant or what it could do, in spite of my efforts to train them and in spite of the fact that these people were spiritual and intelligent. Holding back from the energy exchange seems to short-circuit the capacity to appreciate Reiki. For this reason, I suggest asking anyone you attune to fulfill the same energy exchanges—such as giving energy to help heal the earth and to create a better, more peaceful world—mentioned in the sections of this book where Reiki attunement chants are provided.

The Healing Attunement Process

There is a variation of the attunement process, called a healing attunement, that you should know about as well. It does not involve actually attuning a person to Reiki. Instead, a person is empowered with a blast of healing energy that is often very helpful. To perform a healing attunement, do the same process as for a First Degree attunement, except for a few minor changes. You will first of all intend that the attunement is a healing attunement, and intend it toward a specific issue or illness, if necessary. Then draw the six symbols in the air while contracting the perineum muscle and lifting the tongue to the roof of the mouth. Blow the violet breath into the crown chakra, and guide it all the way to the base of the spine. Then draw out the Usui Master symbol over the person's head, and guide it visually all the way to the base of the spine. Repeat this process with Cho Ku Rei, without raising the person's hands over his or her head. Repeat again with Sei He Ki. Finish this process with Hon Sha Ze Sho Nen.

Come to the front of the person and blow over the person's chakras from top to bottom and back up to the top. Then move behind the person, place your hands on his or her shoulders, and three times mentally say: *May Divine love and wisdom empower this Reiki healing attunement.*

Then place your hands at the base of the person's skull, visualize three Cho Ku Rei symbols sealing the process by going into the brain, and say: *I now seal this process with Divine love and light.*

Then return to the front of the person and blow a final healing blessing to him or her while releasing the perineum and tongue.

A healing attunement can be for physical issues, mental issues, or even just helping a person in dealing with daily life.

What Comes Next

Knowing now how to pass an attunement for each degree of Reiki, and having been attuned to all three degrees of Reiki, you may feel like the journey is over. But in fact the journey has just begun. What comes after these pages is new and groundbreaking information: uses of Reiki that transform consciousness and change the understanding of what Reiki is. The following information is new even to most fully trained Reiki Masters.

18

Sahu Reiki

I was attuned to Third Degree Reiki in 1995. During that year, I spent much of my time living in a tent at the Omega Institute for Holistic Studies in Rhinebeck, New York. Many of the people who came to work for the summer lived in tents, and as one of them, I had to give up my usual practice of burning candles at my spiritual altar every evening as I do when I am at home. To make up for this absence in my life, I began experimenting with using Reiki in ritualistic ways, synthesizing Reiki with esoteric practices that were part of my spiritual life.

Reiki and Egyptian Metaphysics

Since a large part of my spiritual path involved working with the Egyptian Goddess Sekhmet, I began utilizing Reiki in the framework of Egyptian metaphysics. Eventually I was made aware that the Sahu, which is the most Divine aspect of the human being, an energy body that essentially exists outside of time and space, can be attuned to Reiki. Even though it is not physical, it can be attuned. It can also send attunements if attuned to Third Degree Reiki. How this is done will be explained later.

Temporary Attunements for Healing

Hon Sha Ze Sho Nen, like the Sahu, seems to be beyond time and space, or at least able to transcend them. Through accidental experimentation, I came to discover that when these two forces are brought together, both with the capacity to transcend time and space, they make it possible for Reiki attunements to be released or energetically turned off.

Normally a Reiki attunement lasts for life and cannot be taken away once it is given. The advantage in having the capacity to perform an attunement that is temporary is that one can attune parts of the body, areas that are diseased or in need of intensive healing, to Reiki. One would not do this under the normal limitations of Reiki, since normally a Reiki attunement cannot be released. For example, to attune a person's liver to Reiki in the old way would be to have the liver flowing Reiki for the rest of the person's life. This would become overwhelming for the person and perhaps even frightening. (I know this from experience, as I once attuned a vertebra after an injury I suffered, and it flows Reiki constantly. I eventually became used to it, but it frightened me at first.)

How can the attunement be released? Because the attunement comes from a place that can transcend time and involves a symbol that can transcend time, the issue of time becomes irrelevant. When an attunement is given from a person in a physical body, the body is rooted in the time/space matrix. Therefore any attunement that originates through the person's body is subject to the limitations of that matrix. In the time/space matrix, something that is energetically supposed to last for a lifetime will last a lifetime. But when the attunement is given from outside of time, it is not subject to the same laws, even though the person being attuned does exist in the time/space matrix. Since the attunement is not given from a particular point in time, that element of the equation is a free and open variable. That open window, so to speak, allows for the possibility of the attunement to be released by the Sahu, and only by the Sahu. Perhaps if I had a better understanding of relativity and the laws of physics I could explain it better.

I do not use this technique when attuning my students to Reiki because I feel that I have no right to release an attunement at a later date. Attunements that are for the purpose of making one a Reiki healer should not involve the Sahu because they should last for a lifetime. The Sahu Reiki methods are only recommended for specific healing issues, such as attuning a person's cancer to Rish Tea Reiki or attuning a person's lungs to Reiki when they have pneumonia. To use the Sahu Reiki method of attunement for attuning someone as a healer would be unfair, leaving them with the fear that this ability could be taken away at any moment by the teacher. Such a dynamic is not only unfair; it is also unwise.

Perhaps the best way for you to understand how Sahu Reiki works, and the new awareness it brings to Reiki and to life, is to experience it. My theory on why Sahu Reiki works the way it does is based on intuition and guesswork. But my experiments with Sahu Reiki have resulted in methods that can manifest profound healing. The techniques do work and are highly recommended.

The Sahu Attunement Process

Soon you will be using the chant to be attuned to Reiki at the Sahu level for all three degrees of Reiki. Though the Sahu can release attunements, this attunement is being sent to your Sahu from me, in body, using the chant as a vehicle to deliver the attunement. An attunement given in such a manner to the Sahu cannot be released, even though it will empower the Sahu to be able to give attunements that can be released. This is because as a teacher, I cannot see having the right to release this attunement. Therefore, a Reiki attunement is being sent by part of me that exists in time/space to part of you that exists outside of time/space. Once that part of you is attuned, you will have the ability to release Reiki attunements that are given from that part of you that exists outside of time/space. You will not be capable of releasing attunements that you have given from traditional means, nor will future attunements given in traditional fashion be influenced by this attunement of your Sahu. There is a separate technique that will empower you to send Reiki attunements from your Sahu once it has been attuned.

Just as with all other Reiki attunements, you will need to think of an appropriate energy exchange for this attunement. I suggest sending a total of twenty-four hours of Reiki toward ending world hunger. Such an energy treatment works by changing the ways we think, thus changing the economic and political realities that lead to hunger and starvation.

You can, of course, do any other act of good works that feels right for you at this level of energy exchange.

Remember, set a day that feels special to you for receiving the attunement. Take a sea-salt bath to clear your aura. Go to a place that is sacred to you. If you wish, light candles to Dr. Usui and the Divine. Ask for the attunement by reciting the following chant.

Blessed be the Ones who brought us Reiki
Blessed be the Ones who continue this sacred light
I ask that my Sahu be attuned to Reiki
For First, Second, and Third Degree
Blessings unto all
Blessings unto me

Celebrate this day as you wish, for how you view the universe will forever be changed with the use of this new ability with which you have been gifted.

19

Sending and Releasing Attunements

Sending and releasing Reiki attunements through the Sahu is perhaps the most complex aspect of Reiki to understand in theory, and yet perhaps the easiest aspect of Reiki to practice. Let me explain a little about how I came to discover the uses of Sahu Reiki.

How I Discovered the Sahu Method of Reiki Attunement

As I mentioned previously, the Sahu is the most Divine aspect of the human in Egyptian metaphysics. It is our energy body that is almost Godlike. In working with the Goddess Sekhmet, I was told that if I visualized a golden light coming down from my Sahu, through my mouth, and down into the earth, and imagined all words that I spoke coming out of and being formed by that golden light, that it would activate the energy of my Sahu in all that I spoke. In other words, I was given a means to perform Hekau, or magical words of power. I would use this technique only when performing the most sacred magical rites.

One of the things that I found interesting was this relationship between the breath and sacred energy. I was using the violet breath in Reiki attunements, and I was using the golden breath of my Sahu to invoke its powerful energies in my spiritual practice. As one who likes to experiment, I wondered what it would be like to attune my Sahu to Reiki and see what changes might occur for me as a spiritual being. I never thought it would lead to being able to release attunements.

The Sahu Method and the Hekau Technique

I attuned myself to Reiki at the Sahu level by holding out my hand and consecrating it to represent my Sahu, then performing an attunement on it just as I would a stone or other object. I immediately attuned my Sahu to all three degrees of Reiki. As I figured, my Sahu was more than capable of handling the shift. I felt a little light-headed, but nothing more than a usual Reiki attunement.

Through experimenting with the Hekau technique, I discovered that I could request my Sahu, which was now attuned, to send Reiki or to attune things on its own. I tried this with stones at first, holding a stone in my hand and using Hekau to ask my Sahu to attune it to Reiki. I could not simply ask, but had to ask using the Hekau technique I had learned to communicate with my Sahu, visualizing the golden light coming down from my Sahu into my mouth and down to the earth. The phrase that worked best for me, and the one I suggest you use for working with your Sahu, is:

> *By the power of the golden light within*
> *By the power of the sacred breath*
> *I manifest this truth*
> *I now will my Sahu to attune (name) to (Reiki level) Reiki*
> *Now*
> *So be it*

Immediately after saying this, I would blow three times, visualizing the golden words I just spoke going out into the universe and becoming manifested at all levels. It does not seem to work unless I do this. The three breaths activate the statement and give it power. Saying the statement without blowing three times is like using Sei He Ki without empowering it with Cho Ku Rei. In other words, nothing happens unless you do this.

Try using this technique now and see how it works. Find a stone or other object that would be in alignment with being attuned, and use the Sahu method of Reiki attunement. Once the object is attuned, try releasing the attunement by simply saying:

> *By the power of the golden light within*
> *By the power of the sacred breath*
> *I manifest this truth*
> *I now will my Sahu to release the attunement of (Reiki Level) Reiki*
> *that was just sent to (name)*
> *Now*
> *So be it*

Finish this technique by blowing three times to activate what has been said. If you want to think of it like a metaphysical email to your Sahu, think of the three breaths as hitting the button to send it. Until you do, it is not activated.

If you wish, try this several times, attuning an object and releasing the attunement. Hold the object once it is attuned so you can feel Reiki flowing out of it. The amazing thing is measuring this with your own sense of touch, feeling Reiki coming out of a stone, and then suddenly stop coming out, and then coming out again simply due to your requests made to your Sahu.

Using your Sahu to attune things is as valid as the traditional means, as long as you are not attuning a person as a healer in this manner. To do so would be to give you an unfair advantage of being able to release the attunement. It would give you a power over that person that no one should have. The only way that I can see Sahu attunements being valid in such a situation would be in the case where people cannot decide if they want to be attuned for life or not. In such cases, I think it is fine to tell them that you will attune them for a day, week, month, whatever the time frame, and then release it at an agreed upon time. This would allow them the capacity to feel Reiki flowing through their own body. But they would not get the full Reiki experience on a psychological and spiritual level until being traditionally attuned and making the proper energy exchange. This understanding would have to be conveyed to the person as well.

The Most Important Use of Sahu Reiki
The most important use of the Sahu Reiki method of attuning and releasing attunements is for direct healing of organs that need intensive

Reiki. The next time you have a chest cold, attune your lungs to Reiki and notice how your recovery rate speeds up. I have even tried attuning an illness-causing virus or bacteria in my body, and have found that in doing so the illness clears up quickly. Essentially the agents of disease are being turned into millions of little healers in your body. One could argue that this might be against the free will of the virus or bacteria. But, as much as I like to honor free will, my body is my temple and I have final say on what goes on inside of it. I have noticed that when I attune a virus or bacteria, I often suddenly become aware of psychological issues that might be at the root of a disease. So I am not avoiding anything by dealing with the illness in this manner. I am only speeding up the healing process and using inventive means for getting Reiki directly to the source of a health problem.

Investigate your own healing with Sahu Reiki. If you are lucky enough to have absolutely no health issues to be concerned about at the present, try sending an attunement into the past. This is interesting in itself because even though the attunement is sent into the past, you will begin to feel it in the present as a vague shift in your memory, as though you remember experiencing something that you are presently sending to yourself in the past. This is what I mean by Reiki changing your consciousness. How time works and appears loses the linear frame in which we often think of it. I cannot describe what time feels like to me now, but it certainly is not linear in the sense that I once understood it to be.

Some good examples of issues to which to send attunements backward in time are significant traumas, broken legs, burns, gashes, or severe illness. These things often seem cleared up, but once you attune that part of your body backward in time, you will feel the shift of negative energy leave you faster backward in time, which seems to open you backward in time to absorb more of the love and light of the Divine. Your being changes with such uses of Sahu Reiki, even though the issues themselves seem to have had closure. By affecting past time with healing, present time seems to become more open than before. Again, words do not really do justice to this. It is something you must experience and feel to really understand.

Time and Reiki

Questions about time and Reiki are best expressed through my own experience. When I attune part of myself backward in time twenty years, I will also feel Reiki flow through that part of me in the present, unless I specify a time of release during the initial attunement. (How to do this will be shown later.) If I release it five minutes later, does that mean that the Reiki flowed through me for twenty years and five minutes? I do not think this is the case, at least not according to what my body tells me. What my body tells me is that in attuning myself backward in time, the energy of the whole time line of that experience is shifted in the present. So, if I release the attunement after five minutes, the time line of twenty years flowed Reiki for five minutes. To adjust to this, I specify a date or time of release of the attunement when I send it. So, for example, I will attune my lungs backward in time, asking that the attunement be released backward in time at a particular date. In some cases, I might ask that the attunement last for a year, backward in time. Now that time line is programmed to emit Reiki through me during those points in time for eternity. This is because I am not releasing the attunement as a whole. I am simply saying, attune to Reiki this part of my body along these points in time. I will feel shifts in my body in the present, but since the attunement is set to be released before present time as I experience it, I do not feel Reiki flowing through me in the present in that part of my body that has been attuned. Again, analogy and guesswork only touch upon what this is like. I hope someday science will really investigate these concepts and see how Reiki flows through time, what its effects are, and many other important matters.

Practice this on yourself. A general exercise that may work for all people would be to attune your spine to Reiki for the first year of your life. This is just to experiment with the energy and see how this technique works. It does not matter if you were ill or not. And as a fan of chiropractic, I believe that we always carry some degree of emotional tension in our spines that can be released for our well-being. To do this, simply say the following chant.

By the power of the golden light within
By the power of the sacred breath
I manifest this truth
I now will my Sahu to attune my spine to First Degree Reiki
On the day I was born
And to release this attunement backward in time
On my first birthday
Now
So be it

Blow three times to activate the attunement. You will probably experience an emotional release upon doing this. I feel energy clearing out of my spine now having performed this experiment during the writing of it. It is as if a tunnel of light has moved through my spine to open me, but that this is being felt in the present from an action in the past. My perspective is that this healing continues through the rest of your life.

It works like this: right now your spine has been attuned for the first year of your life, which you have been able to absorb for only a few minutes. A year from now, your spine will have been attuned for the first year of your life, a healing that you have been able to absorb for a year. In ten years, you will have been able to absorb the healing for ten years. The healing itself is constant now along that time line, unless you tell your Sahu to release the attunement as a whole. Though there is no reason to do this, you can do so by simply using the Hekau technique to release the attunement you just sent out.

By using these Sahu Reiki methods, you will come to actually sense and experience time in a way that is nonlinear. You will begin to think of time as fractal geometric points, as patterns that can be woven into and around each other. The straight line of time is an illusion, and Reiki at this level is a practical healing means of helping us see and feel that. What does that mean? It means Reiki at this level helps us to move further along in our own evolution, to be able to start having experiences that are fifth dimensional, where time is like rubber, something that can be twisted, turned, shifted, and changed. This leads to conceptualizing things, thinking about life in entirely different ways. Perhaps, when our language starts to evolve with us into this new awareness, I will be able to give a more thorough explanation of it.

Use this new awareness to promote your own soul healing and physical healing at levels never before dreamed of. For me to give examples at this point only limits your power to imagine for yourself.

This is now your homework, to use this technique to work on yourself. Know as well that it is not only your body that can be attuned for healing. If you attune your bed backward in time for a year, that means you will have slept in a Reiki bed for a year, absorbing all that wonderful energy. I have often attuned food, clothing, rooms, and other items I was in contact with during certain periods of my life. The shifts you feel with this kind of Reiki are profound. And all it takes is asking your Sahu to perform the attunement, and blowing three times. Let your imagination go wild, always remembering to honor the free will of others; do not include them in your healing, or perform healing on them, unless permission is given. In other words, do not attune your bathtub to Reiki backward in time when you were a child because that would affect your whole family. But you can attune all the water that you took a bath in during childhood to Reiki. Always ask, How will the Reiki contact me? Also ask, Will anyone else absorb Reiki because of this? If someone else is involved, you will need permission to perform the attunement in good faith.

20

Reiki in All Things

The common understanding of Reiki is that it is Universal Life Force, and that it will flow out of the hands of people. This understanding is not wrong, however it is quite limited. It leaves one with the feeling that Reiki is simply another name for chi or prana or any other name given to the life energies that radiate out from all living things and that flow through us constantly. Do we really understand what life force is? If examined in a scientific view, what happens on the molecular level with Reiki? Is it simply bringing in more energy of life, the way a thick ancient forest fills every being inside of it with life-force energy? I believe it is doing more than this, and operating in ways that most of us cannot easily comprehend.

Experimentation vs. Tradition

My views about Reiki are based on experiments, not what has been passed down in the oral tradition of Reiki. There is much about that tradition I do not trust, as some information about the history of Reiki seems to have been fabricated. Often the focus of such a history seems to be more about glorifying personalities than about investigating what Reiki truly is. I think it is important to honor Dr. Usui and those who came after him, but let us get on with discovering the many things Reiki is capable of. Right now, the common view of Reiki is quite stiff. Some people in the world of Reiki get upset when I talk about sending Reiki to nonhumans, as if the beauty of this universal energy is reserved for humanity alone. And very few Reiki Masters that I have known advocate experimentation or creative uses of Reiki. Their view is often limited to symbols, hand positions, history (perhaps better known in this case as mythology), and promoting a personal Reiki practice. We have in our hands one of the most beautiful gifts in all creation, and all we can do is think how to make money off it and do some healing.

The experiments that I have done show that Reiki is much more complex than most Reiki Masters are willing to admit. These experiments began before I became familiar with Sahu Reiki. Though Sahu Reiki and attunement chants are certainly new in the eyes of most Reiki Masters, they are but the tip of the iceberg in as far as Reiki exploration can go. What I have discovered in my experiments is that all things have a certain Reiki imprint, a vibration that can be articulated within the Reiki system. This does not mean that all things have the capacity to flow Reiki without being attuned, but does mean that there is the capacity to flow the Reiki of any particular object, being, thought, action, anything that exists or has existed. That is quite a bold statement, but true.

The Divine and Reiki in All Things

Think of the mind of the Divine, that all creation carries something of the Divine within it, that we are all thoughts of the Divine in some sense. This Divine energy never leaves us, and is always part of who we are. If it did leave us, we would not exist. The Divine is eternal, going beyond death and the limitations of time and space. So even in the death of a being, object, action, or thought, the Divine spark lives on. The Divine spark that is in the sheet of paper on which these words are written will exist forever, even after the sheet of paper is long gone millions of years from now. One can be attuned to these Divine sparks, which have their own unique vibration. In other words, there is Reiki in all things, and the attunement process is what allows us to open up to this energy. Since the Divine is eternal and infinite, attuning yourself to the Reiki of another being does not take away from the Divine spark existing in that being. Nothing can take away from it, for it has no end.

Redwood Reiki

These are not simply metaphysical theories. I began this experiment in 1996 in a redwood grove north of San Francisco. It occurred to me to try to incorporate the energy of a redwood tree into a Reiki attunement.

I stood next to a tree and consecrated my hand to represent myself, and by performing the attunement process over my hand, I attuned myself to Redwood Reiki.

This was done simply by pinching from the aura of the tree during those times in the attunement process when I would normally add an alternative symbol into the attunement process. I would pinch energy from the aura of the tree, and guide it into my hand just like one of the symbols. What occurred for me was profound and amazing. I began to feel as if I was part redwood. The energy that flowed out of my hands when I asked to flow Redwood Reiki was strong and beautiful and full of a loving power I had only felt before when being with these trees. The attunement lasted, and I can still flow Redwood Reiki at will. Since there is no symbol for this, I simply visualize a redwood tree as the symbol, and chant "Redwood Reiki" in combination with using Cho Ku Rei.

The Attunement Process

This probably sounds pretty far out and unbelievable. Again, let your own experience guide you. Tune into any plant, tree, or other object that feels in alignment with what you are seeking and ask if that being is willing to work with you on this level.

Now stand next to that being. Blow over one of your own hands and ask for that hand to represent you during the attunement process. You can visualize the tips of your fingers being your head, your palm as your abdomen, and so on. Now perform the attunement process for First and then Second Degree Reiki, each time pinching energy from the aura of that being that you are asking to be part of this attunement. Guide in each pinch as you would an alternate symbol in the attunement process. When you have finished both First and Second Degree attunements in this process, hold your hands against your heart and abdomen and flow the Reiki of that being that you just attuned yourself to by visualizing the being as a symbol, chanting the name of it, and following with Cho Ku Rei. Notice the vibration in your hands and how it is different from Reiki in the sense of Reiki as it is typically taught. You will notice a distinct energetic imprint of the Reiki of whatever it is you have just attuned yourself to, an energetic imprint that suggests the presence of that which you have attuned yourself to, being alive and vibrating within your own hands. For example, when I flow the Reiki of rose quartz, it almost feels like a piece of rose quartz is in my hands. These experiences might sound very implausible, but only in performing the exercises mentioned in this chapter can you actually understand them sufficiently.

A much simpler way of doing this is simply to ask your Sahu to attune you to the Reiki of whatever it is you wish to be attuned to. That works just as well. But I wanted you to understand the method as it first came to me.

Synthesizing Sahu Reiki with this technique of attuning yourself to the Reiki of a particular being or object is where Reiki truly opens up as a multidimensional healing force. I love using Redwood Reiki for the feeling of it, and I am sure that I get healing from using it. But what about the capacity to use this form of Reiki to access the energies of herbs, crystals, stones, and other medicinal energies that can be manifested as Reiki?

Some Experiments

Here's a good experiment to try. Take a normal river stone or simple rock, and ask your Sahu to attune it to the energies of rose quartz, which can be used for healing the heart chakra. Once you have attuned the stone, place it over your heart and feel the Reiki flowing into you. Notice the difference between this and normal Reiki.

Try taking a bath and attuning the water to the Reiki of red roses.

Try attuning a glass of water to the Reiki of your favorite meal, and then drink it. You will not actually taste the meal, but you will feel a vibration in the water that resonates so strongly that you might think you are tasting the meal.

You are limited in this use of Reiki only by the power of your imagination, honoring free will, and using common sense. Experiment with the world around you, realizing you have access to the Divine spark that is in all things, that the Divine really is everywhere and accessible. The concept of a silent invisible God who will not speak to us is an illusion. The Divine is willing to show itself in these Divine sparks as Reiki flowing through your hands.

Again, I strongly advocate experimenting, though be careful of what you attune yourself to. This is a powerful technique that can be used for all kinds of healing work. Once when in Mexico, I was swimming in the ocean and became trapped in a strong back tide behind some rocks. The only way I could get out was to let the ocean tumble me over the rocks. I came out of the ocean bloody, bruised, and with a back injury. I was used to being able to adjust myself through body movements that my body learned while under Network Chiropractic care, an alternative type of chiropractic care that facilitates the body learning to adjust itself. I tried to turn my torso and get the adjustment that would end the pain I was in to happen, but the muscles were too tight and in too much pain to move how I wanted them to move. The pain was severe and went on for hours until I thought of asking my Sahu to attune my back muscles to the Reiki of the drug my dentist used to numb my mouth when filling cavities. My Sahu did this, and my back suddenly stopped hurting, and I was able to move my body so that it adjusted itself, releasing the spinal imbalance that was causing me the pain. Once I adjusted myself, I released the attunement and felt my muscles as normal.

The Medical Potentiality of Reiki

Perhaps the American Medical Association would not approve of my use of Reiki to heal my back, and admittedly there is the chance for this to be used in ways that are not necessarily about healing. But imagine what the advantages would be if research was done on how this actually works on a molecular level. What if drugs for AIDS, cancer, and other diseases could work efficiently simply at the energetic level? This would mean a true revolution in health care across the world. Reiki might hold the key for medicines to be made available in parts of the world where people currently cannot afford modern medical care. Certainly I do not advocate one experimenting with this use of Reiki without being aware of the consequences or without having the right professional training. I used the dental drug on my back in Reiki form because I was in severe pain. I do not understand the pharmaceutical world enough to call myself an expert, nor would I play with these energies at random. I do, however, encourage research in this field by trained professionals who could measure the results and help humanity understand which drugs would work effectively in Reiki form.

I also wonder, when looking at the issue of drug addiction, if it would not be possible to treat addicts with a variable use of Reiki drugs. Would it be possible to lower and release the physical addiction, while keeping the psychological addiction pacified through Reiki form until the psychological issues were dealt with? I do not have the answers, nor do I have the understanding based on research to discuss each particular drug possibility. Perhaps some drugs do not work on an energetic level, but the dental drug I accessed with my Sahu felt entirely like the real thing. This deserves to be researched, and this is one of the most important reasons I have for writing this book and for making sacred knowledge public.

Other issues to be looked at, but which I do not feel personally qualified to investigate, are the reactions of viruses and bacteria when actually attuned to the Reiki of drugs used to fight them. Is there the possibility for accelerated healing at a low cost, perhaps even free?

Other Potentialities for Reiki

What other things might be possible with Reiki? I do know that flowers that are in a vase of water attuned to Reiki will last for an extremely long time, but what impact could this form of Reiki have upon agriculture? Is it possible to regenerate the life force of the land by simply attuning farmland to Reiki or by irrigating fields with water that is attuned to Reiki? Does soil attuned to the Reiki of nitrogen act like a fertilizer? These might seem like far-off fantasy questions, but I believe that one day Reiki will be part of all sciences because it is part of our fifth-dimensional awareness. It is part of our human evolution to a greater spiritual path, one in which the energy of the Divine is recognized and felt openly in all aspects of life.

I was once criticized by a girlfriend who said I was misusing sacred energy by attuning laundry water to Reiki instead of using detergent. However, I believe I was not only helping the planet by not using harmful agents in the water, but that I was also elevating doing laundry to being something of a holy activity, as all aspects of our lives should be. The uses of Reiki in this form are endless, and open the human mind and world into a New Age, one far greater than the one we imagine filled with psychic hotlines and tarot decks. A planet filled with Divine light is the true potential, and Reiki is one means of promoting that reality.

One aspect of this kind of Reiki, for which I have not been given a name or found one, has to do with how different Reiki energies interplay upon one another. One way in which to do this is to repeat the exercise of laying two stones attuned to Reiki on your back. However, in this case you will attune one stone to Yin Reiki and the other to Yang Reiki. Remember, everything has a Divine spark of Reiki that is unique. Just the concepts of yin and yang are enough for an element of Reiki to exist that can be tapped and carry the vibration of these concepts. Yin is receptive and feminine. Yang is assertive and masculine. Each flows into the other to maintain balance. Feel this as the two stones flow Reiki through your spine. I usually put the Yang Reiki stone at the top of my spine and the Yin Reiki stone at the bottom of my spine because traditionally yang is heavenly and yin is earthly. The vibration this brings into your spine is wonderful, a kind of harmony and sense of well-being that two stones attuned to normal Reiki, in most cases, do not quite project.

Now, try holding those same two stones in each hand. Put the Yin Reiki stone in your right hand to balance out your masculine half of the body, and the Yang Reiki stone in the left hand to balance out the feminine side. (The left side of the brain, which controls the right side of the body, has primarily rational functions, which are typically associated with masculine yang energies, whereas the right side of the brain, which controls the left side of the body, has more emotional/artistic functions, which are typically associated with feminine yin energies.) In each case, the Reiki flows toward its opposite. In other words, these energies operate in Reiki form the same way they do when conceptualized. There is a dynamic between them, an interplay that creates an entirely new variable in the healing aspect of Reiki.

Given the dynamic Reiki forces such as this simple exercise demonstrates, how might they be tapped and used in the world of physics and engineering? Is it possible, using dynamic Reiki forces, to create energy batteries that are nothing more than stones programmed to emit this

Divine energy in a particular way? If so, they would be an inexhaustible supply of energy. Perhaps this sounds like science fiction, but later in this book you will be shown ways of running cords of Reiki through time and space by connecting them to Reiki batteries, which keep the cords running Reiki energy through them like little Reiki laser beams. On some level then, the concept of a Reiki battery does work. The issue is, can it be made into something that can power an engine or light a light bulb? When this ability is discovered, the whole of our world will be radically changed by it.

21

Reiki Cords

Hopefully by now you will have practiced using Sahu Reiki enough times to be proficient using it. Your awareness of time/space and the energies that flow through us and around us has probably shifted quietly away from what your awareness was before you came into contact with this book. Most people think Reiki is something that flows only out of human hands, and only when directly attuned by a Reiki Master in person. Here you have already had the option of being attuned through chants, exposed to alternate symbols, learned how to send and release Reiki attunements from your Sahu, and tapped into the potential for flowing the Reiki of a tree or stone or concept. All of these things have powerful healing possibilities. For me, however, the supreme component of using Reiki is in being able to manifest a cord of Reiki running through any two points in the time/space matrix.

Sending Reiki vs. Running a Reiki Cord

One could say that sending Reiki is running a cord between two points in the time/space matrix, but this is not true. When sending Reiki, the Hon Sha Ze Sho Nen symbol acts as a portal or vehicle to transport the Reiki to the desired space. The Reiki does not flow in a straight line from point A to point B in such a case. In other words, if you are sending Reiki to a friend across the room using the traditional methods, there is no Reiki path between you. Reiki leaves your hands, and suddenly appears at the destination. It does not actually go through time/space, but simply begins to manifest itself at the desired location. If people walked in between you and a friend to whom you are sending

Reiki, they would not be in the path of the Reiki flow. Though they might feel a shift in the overall energy of the room since Reiki is being sent and received in the same room, they would not feel Reiki flowing directly through them to arrive at your friend. When running a Reiki cord, however, Reiki flows like a laser beam between two points, and anything that comes between those two points is directly contacted with Reiki. How to do this will be explained shortly.

The Healing Benefits of Reiki Cords

There are several healing benefits of using Reiki cords. First, it is possible to run Reiki cords through areas of disease in the body, bringing greater healing potential since millions of cords can be run through a variety of points surrounding the areas of disease. For example, I have often been plagued with earaches. Due to some injuries suffered as a child, water tends not to drain from my ears if I take a bath or go swimming. Because I love swimming and bathing, I have been prone to ear problems much of my life. The water remains and I get ear infections. But once I discovered how to use Reiki cords, I realized that every cell in my ears, inner ear, and the bones surrounding my ears are all potential points through which to run Reiki cords. Now if I feel an earache coming on, I ask my Sahu to attune all the cells of my ear canal to send a Reiki cord to each and every other cell in my ear canal. The cord holds until it is no longer needed. This healing can be expanded by running Reiki cords from the jaw through the ear up into parts of the skull, so that a cord of Reiki runs through the ear near the eardrum and inner ear, where infections can be quite nasty. Since a Reiki cord is like a minilaser, the Reiki flows more intensely than usual. Given that you can run as many cords as you wish between the points surrounding your ear—some small, some large, some at various angles—it is possible to create an entire web of amplified Reiki that flows Reiki continuously until the cords are released. Hence, instead of taking some medication before you go to sleep, it is possible to manifest the Reiki cords around the ear before you fall asleep. When you wake up the next morning, you will find that eight hours of Reiki flowing through you has released the infection.

Such uses of Reiki cords, I believe, would be beneficial especially in the treatment of cancers or other forms of illness where the disease resides in a specific physical area of the body. Once that area is identified, Reiki cords can be manifested immediately to treat the illness.

How to Manifest a Reiki Cord

To practice manifesting a Reiki cord, start by working with stones. I suggest stones because they are usually large enough for you to definitely feel the Reiki flowing from one point to another. Also, you can move them around, place them on your body, in your hands, or elsewhere. This allows you to feel that the cord is running between the stones. And you'll notice that as the stones move, so does the Reiki cord.

Manifesting a Cord in Stones

Using two stones, hold up both and say:

> *By the power of the golden light within*
> *By the power of the sacred breath*
> *I manifest this truth*
> *I now will my Sahu to attune these stones*
> *To be as First and Second Degree Reiki batteries*
> *Manifesting a cord between them*
> *Of First and Second Degree Reiki*
> *Now*
> *So be it*

Remember to blow three times to activate the statement. Once you have done this, the Reiki cord will be manifested between the two stones. You can place your hand in between the two stones and feel the Reiki flowing. Put one stone at one end of the room and the other at the other end of the room, and place your hand between them. You should still feel the cord. Place a book between them. Move your hand to one side of the book or the other, and notice that the cord of energy goes right through the book.

I was once on an airplane from San Francisco to New York and for the sake of experiment ran a Reiki cord from my refrigerator at home all the way to the can of soda that was sitting in front of me on the pullout table. This was halfway across the United States, and I could feel the cord of Reiki go right through me, back to the refrigerator at home.

As for the terminology, you might ask why you should use the term "Reiki battery" when attuning the stones to run a cord of Reiki between them. When I first developed this exercise, the cord would fade very quickly. I thought that, because concepts and words have a spark of the Divine that can be turned into a flow of Reiki, the idea or concept of a Reiki battery might be enough to maintain the cord. I tried it and it was a success.

Manifesting a Cord in Your Body

Once you have played with using stones to manifest a Reiki cord, try running a Reiki cord through your own body. If you have no illness that needs to be addressed, I suggest working on the spine. Once again, releasing tension from the spine adds vitality and helps you stay in balance emotionally. To run a cord through your spine, simply say:

By the power of the golden light within
By the power of the sacred breath
I manifest this truth
I now will my Sahu to attune my C-1 vertebra and my coccyx
To be as First and Second Degree Reiki batteries
Manifesting a cord
Of First and Second Degree Reiki between them
Now
So be it

Remember to blow three times. Feel the cord of energy running through your spine. You might want to stretch out on a bed and really soak up this intense treatment. When you are ready, release the attunement by simply saying the following chant.

By the power of the golden light within
By the power of the sacred breath
I manifest this truth
I now will my Sahu to release
The attunement of my C-1 vertebra and my coccyx
As First and Second Degree Reiki batteries
And to release any Reiki cords between them
Now
So be it

Blow three times, and feel the energy of your spine return to normal.

One way I use this method is to run Reiki cords through my rib cage when I am congested. The cords go through the lungs, and the intensity of the Reiki clears up the lungs—sometimes in less than an hour.

Treating Others with Reiki Cords

When using Reiki cords in the treatments of others, I get their permission first. It might not always be possible to fully explain what you are doing, but make sure the person understands that energy will be running through the body between certain points, and that it will be more intense than most Reiki treatments. Let the person know that at any point the treatment can stop if it becomes overwhelming or uncomfortable.

Attuning Hands and Objects as Reiki Batteries

You can also attune the hands to be as Reiki batteries, causing them to flow laserlike Reiki between them. I have used this a few times on myself while giving people Reiki treatments, but only with people who are used to intensive energy work. In such cases, I will place my hands on opposite ends of the person's head, torso, legs, or wherever I want to focus the treatment, allowing the intensive flow of Reiki between my hands to work on whatever area it is that needs the intensive healing. If I cannot reach my hands so that they are on both sides of the person, I look around the room and attune an object directly across from me to be another Reiki battery. For example, when sending intensive Reiki to a person's heart, I have attuned the massage table right beneath their heart to be a Reiki battery, running a cord of Reiki through the person's heart to my hands. When doing this, I do not feel Reiki flow through me. It is as if the energy suddenly exists on its own between the two points. And even though my hands are part of the equation, I never feel as if the Reiki is flowing through me. It simply exists between whatever two points are named as Reiki batteries.

Running Cords through Time

Another aspect of using Reiki cords is adjusting the Reiki batteries to be at different points in time. I have only done such healings on myself, and have never used them in a hands-on treatment on another person. But running cords through time does work, and it can be a consciousness-expanding experience. In fact, you can go a little too far with this and I caution you not to do anything that you think you cannot handle. But when used wisely, it can be a very effective treatment.

To practice running a Reiki cord through time on your own, I suggest first working with only your own body. Do something simple. Run a Reiki cord of One Love Reiki through your own heart, such that it runs from the day you were born to the present. This is different than attuning your heart to One Love Reiki on the day you were born and releasing it in the present. A Reiki cord is more direct, more intense, and carries with it a signature of awareness, like a psychic reading between the two points. When doing this myself, I have a sudden and very clear awareness of myself on the day I was born. You may or may not experience this, but be prepared for the possibility. To manifest the cord, simply repeat the following:

By the power of the golden light within
By the power of the sacred breath
I manifest this truth
I will my Sahu to attune my heart backward in time
On the day I was born
To be as a First and Second Degree Reiki battery
And to attune my heart in present time
To be as a First and Second Degree Reiki battery

Running a cord of
First and Second Degree One Love Reiki in between
Now
So be it

Remember to blow three times to activate the statement. Allow yourself a quiet space to enjoy this treatment, perhaps doing it just before going to bed or while taking a bath. Feel this love energy zooming through your heart and through time. As you do this, notice what you feel about yourself. What kinds of shifts occur in your consciousness while you are in this treatment? When you are ready, release the cord by saying the following:

By the power of the golden light within
By the power of the sacred breath
I manifest this truth
I now will my Sahu to release the attunements of my heart
As a First and Second Degree Reiki battery
On the day I was born and in present time
And to release the Reiki cord running between these points
Now
So be it

Blow three times to activate the statement. Then notice how the energy in your body returns to normal. You may, however, notice a signature or trace of this experience in the cellular memory of your body.

It will fade fairly quickly, but is enjoyable to pay attention to and notice as a physical reminder of the multidimensional experience you just had.

General Use of Reiki Cords

When using Reiki cords in general, simply identify the points that are to be the Reiki batteries, asking your Sahu to attune them as Reiki batteries and to run a cord of Reiki between them. To release any such attunement, ask your Sahu to release the attunement of the Reiki batteries and to release the Reiki cord. Experiment with this on your own healing path. I have found that running cords through an illness can be a highly effective means of treatment. These cords can be through time or just physically running through the illness in present time. In either case, simply identify the desired target for the Reiki cords and attune Reiki batteries surrounding that target to run Reiki cords between. It's that easy. When ready to release the attunements and the cord, you can ask your Sahu to release them. Use wisdom in all aspects of this work, as the intensity of it is far beyond what many are used to, even those who are extremely familiar with energy work.

22

Reiki Crystals

Some Reiki Masters have investigated integrating crystal work with Reiki. Grids are formed with crystals that are charged to Reiki, and the grid is used to amplify Reiki and aid in healing work or manifesting work. Diane Stein mentions them in her excellent book *Essential Reiki,* and other Reiki Masters are familiar with the concept. As I do not intend to duplicate what you can find in the teachings of Ms. Stein, and have my own separate ideas about Reiki crystals, I will not explore Reiki crystal grids in this writing. However, I do encourage you to look at her book and become familiar with what she has to say on Reiki crystal grids and other interesting aspects of Reiki.

Integrating Crystal Work with Attuned Crystals

What interests me is integrating crystal work with attuned crystals, and having them send Reiki to particular issues in your life. Again, as with much of this book, many will say this is impossible. But just as a candle can be programmed to send Reiki, so can a crystal. The reason that I have put this chapter after the ones on Sahu Reiki is that Sahu words-of-power methods can be used to contact the crystal and literally tell it what to send Reiki to.

Programming Crystals

To work with this concept, one first needs to know about programming crystals. Most students of Wicca and other magical spiritual paths probably have some idea already how this works. A crystal first must be clear of any previous intent that may have been put into it. To clear a crystal, you can immerse it in sea salt for twenty-four hours, hold it under cold running water for about thirty seconds, or smudge it with the smoke of the sage plant. All of these techniques work, and I can vouch for each of them personally. Once the crystal is clear, it can be programmed for a specific intent. Often these intents are for things such as healing, abundance, or empowerment. And in such cases, the crystal might be worn by the person using it or placed on a sacred altar, where the magic is part of some greater spell.

Crystals do emit energy, a concept with which those who make watches run by quartz crystals are quite familiar. Quartz crystals are the kind I most frequently use, and what I recommend. In magically programming the crystal, the energy is focused to do a particular job, as mentioned previously. In Reiki, an attuned crystal can be programmed to send Reiki toward a particular person, issue, or situation.

To program a crystal for the intent of sending Reiki, attune it first to both First and Second Degree Reiki by asking your Sahu, as explained in chapter 19. Then clear the crystal using one of the methods mentioned above. Once the crystal is clear, hold it over your power center, just above your belly button. Visualize the crystal as a friendly mini-sized Reiki healer, which is exactly what it now is. (Since it is like a friend, you should tune in to the crystal and ask for a name by which it would like to be called in your interactions with it.) Then state your intent out loud to the crystal by saying the following: *I do now program this crystal to send Reiki to whatever I ask, whenever I ask.*

Then blow on the crystal to seal your intent.

Whereas most crystals that are programmed for a magical purpose have to be recharged from time to time, I have found that Reiki crystals do not. Perhaps this is because they are really only directing the Reiki flow. Since the Reiki does not come from them, their own energy source is not drained or diminished by the sending of Reiki. (Humans can be drained by flowing too much Reiki, but this is more due to physical and psychological constraints than any real depletion of energy. We are sometimes affected by the energy so profoundly that too much of it flowing through us can be overwhelming. This is apparently not the case for crystals.) I have one crystal that has been sending Reiki for me now for over three years to whatever I ask, and it has not had to be recharged or reprogrammed at all.

Sending Reiki with Programmed Crystals

Now that you have a programmed Reiki crystal, think of it as a friend that can send you Reiki anytime, anyplace. My crystal is in storage in San Francisco, and I have not actually seen it in almost a year. But through my Sahu, I can send a cord of energy (not Reiki) to communicate to the crystal my request for Reiki. To do this, I say:

> *By the power of the golden light within*
> *By the power of the sacred breath*
> *I manifest this truth*
> *I now will my Sahu to send a cord to (name your crystal)*
> *And request that it send Reiki to*
> *(name of person or situation)*
> *For (amount of time)*
> *Now*
> *So be it*

I then blow three times to activate the statement. Remember afterward to thank the crystal for the Reiki it has sent. This can be done through the Sahu as well.

Try this for yourself.

Uses of Reiki Crystals

One of my favorite ways to use Reiki crystals is to receive a Reiki treatment from a crystal right when I am going to sleep. It feels wonderful, and I wake up refreshed because the treatment didn't end as soon as I dozed off. It continued for as long as the crystal was requested to send it.

You can even attune a crystal to Third Degree Reiki and then ask it to attune things for you. Try this yourself, attuning a crystal to Third Degree Reiki and then asking it to attune a stone or other object to Reiki. Make sure that you state the level of the attunement to be sent, and whether or not it will include any alternate symbols. All of your request will be followed exactly as you state, so make sure that you are clear in your request.

Crystals can be used simply as well. You can program a Reiki-attuned crystal for flowing Reiki, and then place it on the body during a treatment. It will be like an extra hand emitting the healing force of Reiki.

One thing I would not do, because I have done it and it made me ungrounded, is to wear a crystal that is attuned to Reiki. The constant flow of Reiki energy can make you ungrounded. If you decide to do this though, do not operate heavy machinery or drive an automobile. Take this advice from one who enjoys experimenting with energy and pushing things to their edge: it isn't worth it in this instance.

The primary advantage of using a crystal instead of sending Reiki yourself is you can use the crystal at times when sending Reiki would be difficult or awkward. Perhaps being at a business meeting in your workplace is not the best place to begin sending a treatment. But if you show up at a business meeting where your full attention is required and suddenly find there is a negative energy in the room that needs immediate attention, you can softly ask your Sahu to contact your Reiki crystal and request a treatment. The treatment will usually start a few seconds after the three breaths activate your request. The three breaths can be so soft that hardly a soul would notice. This is just one example of how having a Reiki crystal can be useful. I'm sure you can and will discover other advantages as you use your own crystal.

23
Reiki Dynamics

I know very little about physics or science. I am a poet and a Reiki Master, not a nuclear engineer or physicist. Much of what I have to say about Reiki dynamics is based on experiments and intuition. It might sound like science fiction, but it is based on reality. I know things that could open doors in the scientific world, that could even manifest something of a Reiki utopian world. What I can do is say what I have experienced, and give insights to what I have imagined during these experiments, pointing toward directions that those more trained than myself can pursue.

The Interplay of Reiki Energies

When I speak of Reiki dynamics, I am referring to the interplay of different Reiki energies upon each other, and how sometimes this interplay creates a force of energy that is more than the sum of its parts. This can best be felt when using Yin Reiki and Yang Reiki flowing through the human spine from different ends of the body. When this occurs, the yin and yang seem to merge into a balanced force that is neither yin nor yang, but is created by them. How this could be used in any scientific realm is going to need to be answered by science, not me.

Scientific Possibilities for Reiki

Given my experiments, what is interesting is what they point to: the possibility of creating energy fields that are inexhaustible and can be altered by changing variables in the equation of what kind of Reiki is being used. These things should be studied at the level of quantum physics. I have attuned electrons and protons to run Reiki cords to each other in each atom in each molecule of water in many of my baths. The sensation of bathing in this is bizarre and probably has no specific healing value at all, but it is entertaining to take a bath in something that is buzzing with webs of Divine light at the subatomic level. But how might this energy technique help us understand how the universe works?

If Reiki and Reiki cords could be measured, it might help in tracking the activity of subatomic particles attuned to Reiki and in analyzing their behavior. Since Reiki cords can be sent through time, this would add an interesting element to the study of physics. What might happen at the molecular level when the atom of one element is attuned to one kind of Reiki and the atom of another element is attuned to a different kind of Reiki? Would this influence the properties of the molecule as a whole? I cannot answer this, but I guess that it might. Can the structure of an atom be changed by running Reiki cords through the quarks and charms, or other subatomic particles that are its very being? Again, this is something I cannot prove or disprove, but think is worth looking at scientifically. Can Reiki, in other words, be the doorway to a scientific alchemy wherein the properties of the elements can be changed or enhanced? We will never know unless this is investigated.

What I feel is the most promising possibility with Reiki dynamics, however, is the chance of creating an inexhaustible supply of energy. The Reiki that flows out of a stone is much stronger than the tingle of energy that one feels when holding a quartz crystal that is not attuned to Reiki. Yet a quartz crystal's energy can be harnessed. Could the energy of a Reiki stone be harnessed as well? If so, how could that energy be amplified through the use of Reiki cords? Can cords running through a stone or other object be affected by other Reiki cords so that there is a layering of energy fields, one surrounding the other or even coexisting so that they meet only at one point of the time/space matrix? Or can they interact more like webs of light?

If I can create webs of light to heal an ear infection, can these same webs provide a source of energy, not in stones but in microchips? Can these chips be programmed to turn Reiki off and on the same way a crystal can, and, if so, can this create an entirely new dynamic of energy that pulsates, has rhythms, and can interact with other fields of energy with different energetic variables but similar magnitudes of strength? What if two chips like the ones I imagine could be programmed to interact so that a third, greater field of energy is created, just as the Yin and Yang Reiki stones create a third energy field when placed on my spine? This should be explored. Perhaps there is a whole field of Reiki technology that can be explored. Let's ask the questions that might lead to this.

Reiki dynamics could influence how energy is conducted through wires. Do copper wires that are attuned to Reiki conduct electricity more efficiently? Reiki has been known to help start electrical items, and I think there is a scientific reason for this. If a copper wire is attuned to one kind of Reiki at one end and another kind of Reiki at another end, will that change how the wire conducts electricity? Is it possible to attune the electrons and protons within a copper wire to run Reiki cords and interact such that a third field of energy flows through the wire on its own so that no electrical source is needed? To what might one attune the electrons and protons in order to manifest this?

Someone with knowledge of how electricity functions might be able to attune electrons to the Reiki of a particular ion or current of energy, while attuning the protons to something entirely different; in theory, their interaction could create a certain third field of energy. If I can make the water buzz with energy with my limited knowledge, what might a trained professional be able to do if attuning electrons and protons to various modes of Reiki and having them interact at the sub-atomic level?

Reiki dynamics could also play a greater part in holistic medicine. In alternative treatments such as acupuncture, how might the Yin and Yang Reiki effect be enhanced to aid in an acupuncture healing session? I knew an acupressure student who would often use methods I have discussed to attune specific acupressure points to run Reiki cords through specific meridians. This technique was often quite effective in her own healing process, and was also effective when she used it on me. How might Reiki dynamics be used to enhance herbal tinctures as well?

These things are speculative, I understand. And there is no study that I am capable of making that will prove or disprove anything. But I can say that having used Reiki to manifest something similar to a biochemical effect on my back when I was injured in Mexico, Reiki does have an effect on the physical world, that vibrations of drugs and perhaps energy fields can be replicated to some degree through Reiki. How exactly that can be used, I leave for the world of science.

Working with Reiki Dynamics

What remains now, however, is the opportunity of taking you into the world of working with Reiki dynamics. I have yet to experience any effect or dynamic of Reiki that is harmful. Sometimes it can be overwhelming, but not directly harmful. For this reason, I feel that exploring this in a book holds no danger.

As before, working with stones is easy and does not cost anything. So, find a stone that is calling to you for this work. Remember, do not just go out and grab any stone you see. Set your intention that you will find the right one. And when you have found the right one, you will know.

Subatomic Attunement of Stones

Once you have your stone, hold it in your hand and ask your Sahu to attune the protons in every atom of that stone to First and Second Degree Yin Reiki, remembering to use the proper wording and to blow three times to activate the statement as revealed in chapter 19. Then feel the stone. Become familiar with what the Yin Reiki feels like.

Once you have done this, ask your Sahu to attune all the electrons in all the atoms in this stone to First and Second Degree Yang Reiki. Then hold the stone and feel the Reiki. It will probably have a certain buzz to it, as if the Yang Reiki and Yin Reiki are flowing into and merging with each other on the subatomic level. But since this merging is infinite, as the Reiki is infinite, the dynamic buzz continues because the two never entirely merge. They are simply constantly flowing into each other.

Now, amplify this buzz by having your Sahu attune all the neutrons in every atom in the stone to be as First and Second Degree Reiki batteries running Reiki cords to each and every other neutron in this stone. Do this by using the Sahu methods discussed in chapter 19. Have your Sahu designate that the Reiki cords are for amplifying all existing Reiki dynamics in the stone. Once you blow that third breath to activate the statement, you will notice a dramatic increase in the buzzing energy of the stone.

How does this work? I do not know, but I must remind you that Reiki is intelligent and of a Divine source. If there is a way to amplify the Reiki dynamic, the intelligence of the Reiki will work toward that in the Reiki cords. Therefore, simply by stating that intention when manifesting the cord helps this become a reality. What actually occurs at the subatomic level at that point is still beyond our capacity to comprehend.

Experimenting with Reiki Dynamics

Experiment with this until you become familiar with the ideas. You should focus on two things. First of all, I use Yin and Yang Reiki because they naturally flow into each other. It is their nature do to so. One could attune the electrons and protons to other forms of Reiki, but they should be forms that will flow into each other, amplify each other, or have some dramatic effect on each other. To attune electrons to One Love Reiki and the protons to Mary and the Three Virgins Reiki would probably make a great stone for healing, but it may not give off a pronounced dynamic. However, let experimentation be your guide.

Second, when focusing the attunement, I like directing them at electrons and protons, because I know this works at a deep subatomic level, and that the Reiki is acting at the core of this material object. But I have also attuned one end of a stone to Yin Reiki and the other half of a stone to Yang Reiki. Then, when holding the middle of the stone, I will feel a very strong interaction between the two. Toward the ends, it will be less so. This is because the Reiki dynamic is occurring most strongly at the border between the two kinds of Reiki as they exist in the stone.

Once you have experimented with stones, try the same experiment on bathwater, and get into the bath. This is so you can feel all the subtle energies that you might not experience in the stone. How does this experience change the way you think about the universe, about the laws of nature? These are important questions, because what Reiki dynamics is really about is collaborating with the Divine to shift and mold creation at the most fundamental level. Again, Reiki cannot harm anything. You are not going to split an atom with Reiki. But you might discover properties in the table of elements that we have never known before, and which can be used for healing and enhancing the human experience.

How might this shift in consciousness affect humanity as a whole? If it was commonly recognized that a magical Divine energy could provide what we now search for in oil, coal, gas, and other energy sources, how might that change our way of thinking as a species? To turn on a light switch in such a circumstance, one would always be aware of a Divine presence, the presence of Reiki that was illuminating the bulb. Daily routine activities would be filled with a constant awareness of the Divine. How could that not change humanity for the better? It would. And it will.

My spiritual guides tell me that what I have stumbled upon is but the tip of the Reiki iceberg, that the very mysteries of the universe can and will one day be explored with Reiki. We have nothing to fear in this. We must go forward into the light and allow for the next stage of human evolution to begin: the capacity to unleash and harness the infinite Divine energy that exists in all things.

24

Reiki as Prayer

In this book, I have tried to emphasize that Reiki is from a Divine Source. Usually in Reiki we try not to label that Source with a name or specific religion. That is because everyone has the right to interpret who or what the Divine is. For some, it may appear with the face of Jesus, and for others it may manifest as Buddha or the Goddess. My own personal belief is that the Divine will manifest itself to you in whatever way you are capable of seeing it. In other words, the Divine is much like a mirror. Those who are angry will see the Divine as angry. Those who are compassionate will see the Divine as compassionate. This is my own interpretation, which allows me to take part in various religions because to me they are all real to some degree. I take pleasure in sending Reiki to the Greek god Pan as much as I do to Jesus, because to me they are both aspects of a multidimensional being far beyond my limited ability to understand within the context of reason and language. But whatever your spiritual path, I suggest incorporating Reiki into it as a form of prayer.

The way this is done is simple. Send Reiki to the Being you see as the Divine. I see this as a way of giving back to the Divine for this beautiful gift of Reiki, as well as the other gifts in life that we receive.

Do this on a daily basis. Not only is it a way of returning this great gift, but it is also a way of direct communion. Once you begin to sense the target of your Reiki while sending treatments, as many of you probably do by this point in your journey, you will be able to sense the Divine directly. There is no journey greater than this, no gift greater than to return the gift and feel the awesome wonder of that Divine Source of all things.

Another way to use Reiki for strengthening your spiritual connection is to send Reiki backward in time to the point of your soul's creation. To feel yourself as you are being formed into an individual consciousness out of the formlessness of the Divine is an experience that carries many gifts and insights. Another way to connect with your overall being and its connection to all things is to run a Reiki cord through time through all of your lives, from the beginning of your soul's creation all the way through to the present. This multidimensional awareness of self is the kind of thing yogis and monks seek for years. You now have that ability within you, wired into your energy field.

But Reiki as prayer does not have to be just about communion with the Divine. Performing acts of good works with Reiki is a means of strengthening your soul and benefiting all things. Remember, Reiki always works for the highest good of all.

Treatments can be sent to your soul directly as well. A soul healing can be one of the most important Reiki treatments you can receive. Simply intend the treatment go to your soul, and use Hon Sha Ze Sho Nen to link the treatment to your soul and the Usui Master symbol version of Diakomyo for soul healing. Cho Ku Rei can be added or not, since the Usui Master symbol works much like a higher version of Cho Ku Rei and does not require empowerment from Cho Ku Rei.

With these tools of Reiki, you have the power to truly walk toward a path of enlightenment in a tangible fashion. You can work toward giving back to the Divine, manifest an awareness of your own beginnings as a soul, perform good works with Divine energy, and send treatments to heal your own soul and mend your own separation from the Divine. Perhaps these are some of the things Jesus meant when He said: "And nothing shall be impossible unto you" (Matt.17:20).

From this point forward, the journey is your own. There are suggested exercises that follow, but how you use Reiki must be guided by your own relationship to the Divine. Listen to this call. There may be some of you who only use Reiki for this one purpose, of returning it to the Divine. And that, in itself, is enough.

25

The Future of Reiki

I feel that Reiki is for all people, something that should be an integral part of the human experience. This does not mean that everyone is going to be or should be a professional Reiki healer, which is a right that is reserved for those who dedicate themselves to the proper training. But let me make an analogy between Reiki and something very common—cooking: not everyone who cooks is a professional chef, yet most people know enough about cooking to feed themselves. So, too, these new tools in Reiki provide a means for most people to feed themselves spiritually, to give healing to their friends and family, and to make Reiki a part of their everyday lives. The simplification of Reiki attunements through chants and working with the Sahu does not diminish the power of Reiki, but only changes how we can access it. We can move forward into new realms of consciousness with this information. I have great visions and hopes for the kinds of advances that could occur by using Reiki in agriculture, medicine, and other sciences, even investigating the potential of inexhaustible energy supplies if Reiki could somehow be tapped the same way electricity is.

Empowering All People with Reiki

If nothing else, this book will empower people to heal themselves. The techniques explored should not be kept esoteric secrets. All people have the Divine right to access the tremendous healing force of Reiki in all aspects of life. We cannot hold back information any longer.

I did, at one point, agree with the view that Reiki was supposed to be an exclusive club that admitted only special people. Those special people were usually, almost always, white upper-middle class seekers of a better way of life. I do not fault them for being in that club. But it is time for the club rules to change so that its membership is not financially exclusive. This book now changes those rules and makes the gift of Reiki accessible to all. I support the tradition in Reiki of maintaining an energy exchange, but not for keeping Reiki in the hands of the few, and especially out of the hands of those who often cannot afford regular health care. True, some people may make the choice to dishonor the energy exchanges suggested in this book with each attunement, but that is their karma with the Divine.

The impact this book will have on the world of Reiki healers is clear. I am sure that eventually society will develop in such a way that there are specialists in Reiki with relationship to all things. Reiki can influence all aspects of our lives, and there may come a day when one goes to a Reiki acupuncturist or a Reiki dentist. I believe there will be farmers who attune their crops to Reiki, and restaurants that will provide food in a manner such that both the food and cookware are Reiki attuned. Because of the information made available in this book, the capacity to bring this Divine energy into every aspect of our lives is now truly limited only by our imaginations. I know with all certainty that professional Reiki healers will remain, but many will have to study harder, deepen their knowledge, and demand more of themselves. They will have to keep up with this energy system as it rapidly evolves. They will need to understand how to use Reiki cords in their practice, how to attune organs and then release those attunements through the Sahu. They will need to know how to integrate Reiki with other forms of energy healing like MAP Coning or VortexHealing® Divine Energy Healing (see Resources, page 145). For even though this book has opened the door of Reiki to many and expanded upon how it could be traditionally used, people will still want to go to a trained Reiki professional who can maintain clear emotional boundaries with a client and perform sessions in a space dedicated entirely to healing.

The world of Reiki healers and the world of Reiki becoming an integral part of all of society can and should coexist. My hope is that many Reiki healers will not only embrace the teachings in this book, but will also embark upon expanding upon them, bringing in new information that is beyond what is written here. This book opens avenues for people to explore deeper possibilities with Reiki. One might become a specialist in using Reiki with animal care, or for plant healing, or in working with medical researchers who will want to investigate Reiki on a deeper level. The uses of Reiki will expand, and as the circle becomes wider, those who have been involved with Reiki for years will have a special place in this transition. If Reiki does become an integral aspect of all society, then I think those who know and understand what Reiki is will certainly have opportunities to use this sacred gift and still support themselves with it.

The Heart of Reiki

Reiki is like the rest of the universe, evolving in ways we often cannot predict. I do not know if Dr. Usui had any idea Reiki would go in the direction it has gone or what Reiki may still be capable of doing. Maybe he did know these things; maybe he knew that no one would be able to understand them one hundred years ago. It doesn't really matter. What matters is that the information in this book is real and true, and it can help humanity. The Divine will continue to provide for those Reiki healers who are in faith with the Oneness of Divine purpose. But the time has come now for this Divine gift to be shared with all who want it. The time has come for this Divine gift to be fully embraced, not just as a way of healing but as a way of living.

When I still believed that Reiki was for those special few, I had already begun my experiments. I kept them secret. I sat quietly at times, knowing that I had knowledge that might help people with AIDS or cancer, but that I was not supposed to violate some invisible law that said Reiki was a stagnant system, an inflexible system, and that it must only be taught in the traditional manner. My consciousness was tortured, and I still did nothing, trying to be true to tradition. I did not change my attitude until working with the spirit of Ra Ta, also known as Edgar Cayce. It was Ra Ta who told me I was supposed to write this book, that this information was not meant for my special little eyes alone, that to keep quiet was antithetical to what the heart of Reiki was all about. And I think that with all of this, we must, as Jesus asks us to do, look at the heart of the law. What is the heart of Reiki law? Does it want an exclusive club that gives the affluent the feeling of being special in the eyes of God, or is it to be used for healing the planet, helping children in ghettos get health care, helping us all see how present and available the Divine really is? Isn't that the real law of Reiki?

As the Reiki circle expands, as it must, Reiki will naturally become more about being connected to the Divine and creating a more democratic and peaceful world. As the Reiki world shifts from being an aristocracy to a democracy, we will see the true power of this force in all aspects of our lives.

Appendix of Exercises

THESE EXERCISES WERE created to make the teachings in this book "user-friendly": to enable you to use the teachings on a daily basis and to incorporate these techniques in your daily life. Some of the exercises may appeal to you more than others. Use what works for you.

Reiki Exercise for Healing a Sore Throat

This technique is highly effective. It works by running Reiki cords through the throat, literally creating an "X" of Divine healing light in the middle of your throat. To do this, simply ask your Sahu to attune the left half of your jawbone to be as a First and Second Degree Reiki battery, and also to attune the right side of your collarbone to be as a First and Second Degree Reiki battery. Ask your Sahu to run a Reiki cord of First and Second Degree Reiki between those two batteries. Now repeat the same process using the right half of your jawbone and the left half of your collarbone as Reiki batteries, and run a Reiki cord between them as well. By doing this, you have created two Reiki cords running through your throat, like an X. The Reiki cord will intensively treat a sore throat. (In fact, I created this exercise only an hour before this writing because I was suffering a dry, painfully scratchy throat. Now, as I write this, the soreness is gone.)

Reiki Exercise for Releasing a Bad Day

You can actually use this for releasing a bad day, week, month, or whatever length of time you desire. It is not the day itself that is being released, but the negative vibrations that are trapped in your energy field through the time/space matrix during that time period. To do this work, you must identify when the negative energy started. You do not need an exact time. You can pinpoint it as an action, state of mind, or whatever, but you do need to identify some starting point. The starting point should not be confused with the cause. What you want is a point on the time line where you can anchor a Reiki battery, and it is best to do it when the negativity started.

Once you have pinpointed the staring point, ask your Sahu to attune your body backward in time to be as a First and Second Degree Reiki battery. Then ask your Sahu to attune your body to be as a First and Second Degree Reiki battery in present time. Now ask your Sahu to run a cord of First and Second Degree Reiki in between those two points.

Your body between those points in time becomes almost like a tunnel of light that intensively pushes out the negative energy you absorbed during that specified time frame. As this tunnel of light pushes the negativity out, your consciousness in present time begins to shift. The time frame no longer seems so bad. So, by changing your own energy field during that time frame, you have shifted your awareness of that time frame into one that is more in line with wholeness.

When you are ready, ask your Sahu to release the Reiki battery attunements and Reiki cord.

Reiki Exercise for Finding Lost Items

This exercise works best on items that are not too small or thin. It works by asking your Sahu to attune the object to be as a Reiki battery, and then attune your heart to be as the other Reiki battery. Ask your Sahu to run a Reiki cord between the two points. Then follow the energy of the cord as it runs through your body, and go in that direction. Use your hand to monitor the cord as it leaves your body to hone in on the lost item.

If an item is too small or thin, the Reiki cord might be too small or thin to detect. If that happens, try doing something to amplify the cord, using your understanding of Reiki dynamics. Usually you will be able to detect the location of the lost item. Of course, this exercise may be more difficult if the item has been lost somewhere other than your own home, but even then it can sometimes lead you to the place where your item can be recovered.

Reiki Exercise for Cleansing the Digestive Tract

The cleansing I mention here is an energetic one. It is not the same as a colonic and should not be treated as the replacement for one. If you have impacted fecal matter, this is not going cure you. What this exercise does do, however, is clear the energy of your digestive tract internally. It is quick and effective. Simply ask your Sahu to attune all fecal matter that has passed through you backward in time to First and Second Degree Reiki at the moment it entered your body as food. The attunement is sent out in mass to all food you have ever eaten, and attunes those atoms and molecules that are part of everything you have eaten that is not absorbed into the body. You will immediately feel a clear lifting of the energy in your whole digestive tract. This helps clear out negative energies or negative thought forms that may be lingering inside of you—or that may have been lingering inside you for years.

Remember, you are what you eat. This includes the vibrations in your food and the thoughts surrounding food when it is made, served, and eaten. Learning to clear your digestive tract of these unwanted energies can help you become clearer both mentally and energetically.

Reiki Bath of Love and Light

This one is exactly like it says, a bath of love and light. Simply begin by filling your bathtub with water. When it is at the level you wish, ask your Sahu to attune all the hydrogen atoms in the water to First and Second Degree One Light Reiki. Then ask your Sahu to attune all the oxygen atoms in the water to First and Second Degree One Love Reiki. The bath then fills with a web of Reiki that exudes love and light. Soak in it as if you are in heaven, because in a way you are.

Reiki Exercise for a Good Night's Sleep

Valerian is an herb that relaxes the body and mind. In this exercise, you ask your Sahu to attune all your muscles to the Reiki of valerian just before you go to bed. Your muscles will then relax into a deep rest to allow for a deep sleep. Since you might forget to release the attunement when you awake the next morning, have your Sahu program the attunement to last only for a few hours. It does not need to be for the whole time you sleep. To program an attunement in such a way, simply state it as follows:

> *By the power of the golden light within*
> *By the power of the sacred breath*
> *I manifest this truth*
> *I now will my Sahu to attune all the muscles in my body*
> *To First and Second Degree Reiki of the herb valerian*
> *And to release this attunement in (fill in the blank) hours*
> *I manifest this now*
> *So be it*

Naturally you must blow three times as with all other Sahu attunements. Once you have done this, sit back and relax into a wonderful sleep.

Reiki Exercise for Clearing the Mind

You could, of course, do a treatment on yourself with the Sei He Ki symbol to clear your mind and have that work. But often you are not in the place to do a treatment. In that case, this exercise can provide some comfort.

Ask your Sahu to attune the inside of each half of your skull to be as First and Second Degree Reiki batteries, sending a Reiki cord of Sei He Ki or One Light Reiki between them. The cord now runs right through your brain, bringing in the necessary illumination to help you find a space of clarity. When you feel clear, release the attunement.

Reiki Exercise for Personal Empowerment

This involves visualizing and internalizing the Cho Ku Rei symbol. It does not involve actually sending Reiki or flowing Reiki, but is about seeing yourself as Reiki, as the power symbol.

Do this exercise while standing. Visualize a large Cho Ku Rei symbol over your abdomen, see it grow, getting bigger and bigger until it fills your whole body. Once you have visualized it growing to fill up your whole body, see it and yourself filling up the whole room, getting larger and larger. Then visualize yourself continuing to grow and the Cho Ku Rei growing with you as if the two of you are merged as one. See both of you growing until you have filled up your whole house or apartment. Allow this feeling of size and power to fill all of your being.

Now see yourself and the Cho Ku Rei symbol growing beyond the size of your dwelling, becoming the size of a city block, and continue growing until you are the size of whatever town or city you live in. (If you live in a rural area, see yourself as the size of the ecosystem around you.)

You can take this exercise as far as you want. Usually, once I am the size of the room, I am feeling pretty powerful. But if you wish, see yourself growing with the Cho Ku Rei to become the size of the whole continent, planet, solar system, or universe if you dare. With the Cho Ku Rei being merged in the visualization of yourself, you are seeing your own Divine power grow, and you become more capable of claiming it.

Reiki Exercise for Expanding Consciousness

My guides tell me that this is something that was used in Atlantis, and is actually used as a doorway by enlightened beings for bilocation. I have never reached that state with it, but I have felt the limitations of time and space slip away.

Like the previous exercise, you will begin by standing. Close your eyes and then visualize yourself as the Hon Sha Ze Sho Nen symbol, seeing it run from your head to your toes. Bring your hands about three inches in front of your third-eye chakra (the middle of your forehead), and hold your hands with your fingers pointing upward to the sky, with your fingertips slightly touching those on the opposite hand. This is somewhat like a prayer hand position, except the palms are not actually touching, just the fingertips. The palms are about an inch or two apart. It is as if you are forming a pyramid of energy with your hands, which, when brought in front of your third eye, opens you to really enter the Hon Sha Ze Sho Nen symbol on a psychic level. This is where the visualization part ends.

From this space, I have been told, you can project your consciousness into any time or place. I have tried it and it works. It is not the same as astral projection. You are not leaving your body or entering a shamanic trance as in a shamanic journey. Your consciousness simply arrives at the destination. Try this for yourself and see.

Resources

Some of the recommended books and websites below may not seem Reiki related, but they are, if we see Reiki as part of a greater whole, trying to create a better, more sustainable world.

For further exploration of Reiki as a professional healer, please read Diane Stein's book *Essential Reiki* (Berkeley, CA: Crossing Press, 1995).

To learn more about working with Devas (Nature Spirits) for self-healing, read Machaelle Small Wright's book *MAP: The Co-Creative White Brotherhood Medical Assistance Program* (Warrenton, VA: Perelandra Ltd., 1990).

To expand your own practice as an energy healer, I strongly recommend investigating VortexHealing® Divine Energy Healing at www.VortexHealing.com.

If you wish to become informed about ways to help heal the planet and live a more sustainable lifestyle, Circle of Life, a nonprofit founded by Julia Butterfly Hill, is an excellent resource. Go to www.CircleofLife.org.

Index

Printed in the United States
by Baker & Taylor Publisher Services

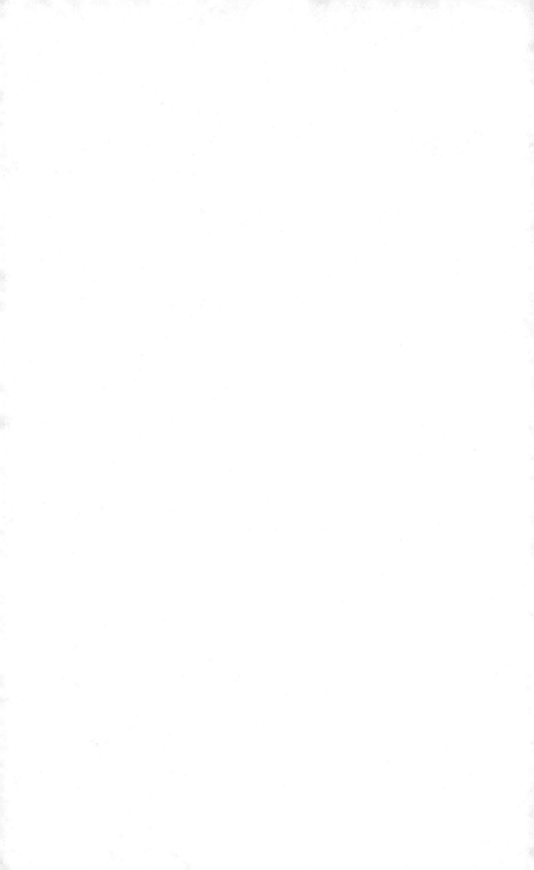